E
on the Western Front

Easing Pain on the Western Front

*American Nurses
of the Great War and the Birth
of Modern Nursing Practice*

PAUL E. STEPANSKY

McFarland & Company, Inc., Publishers
Jefferson, North Carolina

LIBRARY OF CONGRESS CATALOGUING-IN-PUBLICATION DATA

Names: Stepansky, Paul E., author.
Title: Easing pain on the Western Front : American nurses of the
great war and the birth of modern nursing practice / Paul E. Stepansky.
Other titles: American nurses of the great war
and the birth of modern nursing practice
Description: Jefferson, North Carolina : McFarland & Company, Inc.,
Publishers, 2020 | Includes bibliographical references and index.
Identifiers: LCCN 2019051427 | ISBN 9781476680019
(paperback : acid free paper) ∞) |
ISBN 9781476639116 (ebook)
Subjects: LCSH: World War, 1914–1918—Medical care—Western
Front. | Military nursing—United States—History—20th century. |
Military nursing—Canada—History—20th century. | Military nursing—
Great Britain—History—20th century. | Nurses—History—
20th century. | World War, 1914–1918—Participation, Female.
Classification: LCC D629.U6 S74 2020 | DDC 940.4/7573—dc23
LC record available at https://lccn.loc.gov/2019051427

BRITISH LIBRARY CATALOGUING DATA ARE AVAILABLE

ISBN (print) 978-1-4766-8001-9
ISBN (ebook) 978-1-4766-3911-6

Front cover: Allied soldiers on World War I western front
battleground, circa 1915–18 (Shutterstock/Everett Historical);
poster showing a Red Cross nurse holding a wounded
soldier, 1917 (Library of Congress)

———

Printed in the United States of America

*McFarland & Company, Inc., Publishers
Box 611, Jefferson, North Carolina 28640
www.mcfarlandpub.com*

To Deane
Love of this life and all the lives to come

Table of Contents

Acknowledgments

This study grows out of my interest in the history of American medicine, especially the history of primary care medicine in America and Canada in the nineteenth and twentieth centuries. I am deeply grateful to Howard Kushner and the late John Burnham for supporting my return to history of medicine after a three-decade interregnum as a publisher of professional books and journals in psychiatry and psychoanalysis. The DeWitt Wallace Institute for the History of Psychiatry at Weill Cornell has provided a congenial milieu in which to present my work for over three decades, and I remain grateful to the Institute members for their warm encouragement and constructive criticism over the years. In this project I acknowledge the assistance of archivists and special collections librarians and administrators. Their help and guidance, always offered with friendly camaraderie, helped me gain traction in nursing history, a field I turned to late in my career. Specifically, I thank Jean Shulman (American Red Cross), Meg Miner (Special Collections, Illinois Wesleyan University Library), Eric Pumroy and Nicole Joniec (Special Collections, Bryn Mawr College Library), Elisa Stroh (Barbara Bates Center for the Study of the History of Nursing, University of Pennsylvania School of Nursing), Steve Novak (A.C. LongHealth Sciences Library, Columbia University Irving Medical Center), Domenic Tucci (Canadian Nurses Association), and Christine Parsons (Canadian War Museum).

In the search for suitable photos of World War I nursing practice, undertaken principally by my wife and collaborator Deane Rand Stepansky, we acknowledge the kind assistance of Heidi Stover (Smithsonian Institute archives) Jevin Orcutt (American Army Heritage Foundation), George Kutsunis (American Association of Nurse

Anesthetists), Margaret Gurowitz (Johnson & Johnson archives), Simon Jones, historian, and Jon Spence, photographer and grandson of WWI veteran Sawyer Spence of the Queen's Westminster Rifles. Special thanks go to W. Sanders Marble, Senior Historian, Office of Medical History, Army Medical Department Center of History & Heritage, for promptly answering my questions and directing me to relevant sources; David Newman for an astute reading of the manuscript; Nelle Rote for her commitment to World War I nursing studies and enthusiastic support of this project; and Kristopher Spring for expert assistance preparing the final manuscript for submission. The untimely death in 2016 of John Kerr, my gifted colleague at The Analytic Press who, over the years, became a close friend, deprived me of the most discerning reader I have ever had. I am pleased to add my voice to the many who have paid tribute to John, a remarkable editor who placed his enormous erudition at the service of others.

It has been a pleasure working with editorial and production departments at McFarland. My thanks especially to Lisa Camp and David Alff for fielding my questions and suggestions with patience and tact.

On my own home front, the support of my sons and daughters-in-law, Michael Stepansky and Jane Kohuth, and Jonathan and Sy Stepansky, helped keep me on an even keel and provided welcome sounding boards. Additional thanks to Jonathan for helping me along by obtaining books I needed through his university. My grandson Kameron Kohuth Stepansky, bright-eyed and sparkling, uncannily verbal, and fiercely competitive at the chess board from age 5 on, lifted my spirits and helped me put aside books and look to the future. For this, and especially for being my best buddy, I thank him. My brothers David, Bob, and Alan, and their wives, my sisters Debra, Joyce, and Elissa, have provided a bedrock of loving connection over the course of this project and all my projects. Our powerful family bond, which extends to our children, comes from our late parents, Selma and William Stepansky, whose warming glow continues to suffuse our lives. Friends no less than family provided support over the course of this undertaking. My heartfelt thanks to David and Suzie Newman, Keith and Donna Maclellan, Tom and Christine DePoto, Marty and Judy Meyers, Sandy and Pam Harrison, Barbara Wasserman, Annette Miller, Aubree Woods, and Chelsea Woods-Turner.

My wife Deane's belief in the value of my work has been a constant since we found each other at Princeton University in the fall of 1972. In the latter stage of this project, I suffered a loss of near vision, so that her customary role of copyeditor, language consultant, and proofreader was augmented by that of research associate. In addition to reviewing many thousands of photos, she did considerable reading, made notes for me, and urged me to greater clarity of expression. Now, alas, Deane knows far more about nursing in the Spanish-American and Anglo-Boer Wars than any spouse should have to know. Her intimate involvement with the book is a matter of record. What the record cannot convey is the deep and abiding love that underlay her help and the consummate grace with which it was offered and provided. To have as one's partner in scholarship the *cara immortalis*, the immortal beloved, of one's life is a rare and beautiful thing.

Preface

Studies in the history of nursing have their conventions, and this study of American nursing in World War I does not adhere to them. It is not an examination of the total experience of military nurses during the Great War. Excepting only the first chapter, which addresses the American war fever of 1917 and the shared circumstances of the nurses' enlistment, little attention is paid to aspects of their lives that have engaged other historians. I do not review the nurses' families of origin, their formative years, or their reasons for entering the nursing profession. Similarly, there is relatively little in these pages of the World War I nurses as women, of their role in the history of the women's movement, or of their personal relationships, romantic or otherwise, with the men with whom they served.

In their place *Easing Pain on the Western Front* focuses on nursing practice, by which I mean the actual caregiving activities of America's Great War nurses and their Canadian and British comrades. These activities comprise the role of nurses in diagnosis, in emergency interventions, in medication decisions, in the use of available technologies, and in devising creative solutions to treatment-resistant and otherwise atypical injuries. And it includes, in these several contexts, nurses' evolving relationship with the physicians alongside whom they worked. Among historians of nursing, Christine Hallett stands out for weaving issues of nursing practice into her excellent accounts of the allied nurses of World War I, with a focus on the nurses of Britain and the British Dominions. Hallett has no counterpart among historians of American nursing, and as a result no effort has been made to gauge the impact of World War I on the trajectory of nurse professionalization in America, both inside and outside the military.

1

This study begins to address this lacuna from a perspective that stands alongside nursing history. It comes from a historian of ideas who works in the history of American medicine. It is avowedly historicist in nature, grounded in the assumption that nursing practice is not a Platonic universal with a self-evident, objectivist meaning. Rather this type of practice, like all types of practice, is historically determined, with the line between medical treatment and nursing care becoming especially fluid during times of crisis. It is intended to supplement the existing literature on World War I nurses, especially the excellent work of Hallett and other informative studies of British, Canadian, and Australian nurses, respectively. The originality of the work lies in its focus on American nurses, its thematic emphasis on nursing activities, and its argument for the surprisingly modern character of the latter. Close study of nursing practice, especially in the context of specific battlefield injuries, wound infections, and infectious diseases, yields insights that coalesce into a new appreciation of just how much frontline "doctoring" these nurses actually did.

The case for modern nursing practice in World War I is strengthened by comparative historical inquiry that renders the study, I hope, a more general contribution to the history of military nursing and medicine. In each of the chapters to follow, I work into the narrative comparative treatment of World War I nursing with nursing in the American Civil War of 1861–1865, the Spanish-American War of 1898, and/or the Anglo-Boer War of 1899–1902. The gulf that separates Great War nursing from that of wars only two decades earlier, we will see, is wide and deep. In the concluding chapter, I invert the case for modernity by looking forward from America's Great War nurses to the American nurses who served in World War II and Vietnam. If Great War nurses had little in common with the Civil War nurses who preceded them by a half century, they share a great deal, surprisingly, with their successors in Vietnam a half century later.

The focus on nursing practice, then, far from being restrictive in scope, opens to a wide range of issues—medical, cultural, political, and military. Consider, for example, the very notion of healthcare practice, which is determined by a confluence of factors. Specific theories of disease, rationales for treatment of specific conditions, putative mechanisms of cure, and the grounds for "proving" cure are all central to the historical study of healthcare practice. Female nursing practice, with the bodily intimacies it entails, also implicates considerations of gender—of what, keeping to the time frame of this study, early-twentieth-century female hands might do to male bodies, and what the males who "owned" these bodies might comfortably permit female hands to do. Depending on the historical location of nursing practice, issues of social class, nationality, ethnicity, and race may count for as much or more than gender.

By channeling our gaze onto what nurses of the Great War actually did with wounded, suffering, distraught, and dying soldiers, we learn about the many factors that enter into combat nursing at one moment in modern history. The focus on nursing practice provides a new perspective on the medical advances of the Great War; the role of nurses in making and implementing these advances; the new professional status that accompanied this process; and the American military's emerging appreciation of trained nurses, indeed of female officers in general. The focus on nursing practice draws a different picture of the evolution of military personnel policy and the changing social mores and political pressures that accompanied this evolution.

The fate of World War I combat nurses' role back on the home front in the aftermath of war is a separate story that I address but briefly in the concluding chapter. More work should be done on the relationship between military and civilian nursing practice, especially the fate of combat nurses who return to civilian nursing after wartime service. To keep to the subject matter of this study, the experience of America's World War I nurses back in civilian hospitals offers an illuminating window into the frustrations and accomplishments of nurses, indeed of professional women in general, in the American workplace in the two decades between the world wars.

For American readers *Easing Pain on the Western Front* may prove interesting for another reason. Our increasing reliance on nurses to meet the health care challenges of the twenty-first century, especially in the realm of primary care, underscores the relevance of the unsuspectedly modern Great War nurse providers. Indeed, they offer a fascinating point of departure for ongoing debates by nurses, physicians, social scientists, and politicians about the scope of practice of nurse practitioners in relation to physicians. This is because America's Great War nurses, no less than the nurses of other combatant nations, had to step up during battle "rushes" that overwhelmed their surgeon colleagues. At such times, and in the weeks and months of intensive care that followed, they became autonomous clinical providers, true forebears of the nurse practitioners and advanced practice nurses of the present day. The fact that their professional leap forward occurred in understaffed casualty clearing stations and field hospitals on the Western front during the second decade of the twentieth century lends salience to their accomplishments.

Notwithstanding the many streams of contingency that flow into nursing practice at a given moment in history, I hasten to point out that I am not a historian of gender and that my comments on gender, not to mention ethnicity and race, are sparing. I invoke them only in the context of specific nursing activities, especially when they were raised by the nurses themselves. The same may be said of the nurses' personal lives. I ignore neither the emotional toll of combat nursing nor the psychological adaptations to which it gave rise. But here again these issues are addressed primarily in relation to nursing activities, especially the nurses' perceptions of and reactions to the wounded, ill, and dying they cared for. I leave to others more comprehensive study of the gender-related, racial, and psychological aspects of American military nursing in World War I and other wars, noting only that the scholarship of Darlene Clark Hine, Margaret Sadowski, and Kara Dixon Vuic has begun to mine this rich vein of nursing history to great effect.

The cohort of nurses at the heart of this study is not limited to American nurses. They include Canadian and British nurses as well. In the case of the former, the ground for inclusion is not especially problematic, since many Canadian nurses trained in the United States; indeed, some both trained and worked in the States prior to their wartime service. Ella Mae Bongard, for example, a Canadian from Picton, Ontario, trained at New York Presbyterian Hospital, practiced in New York for two years after graduating in 1915, and then volunteered with the U.S. Army Nursing Corps. She ended up at a British hospital in Étretat, where she served with several of her Presbyterian classmates. The Canadian Alice Isaacson, who served with the Canadian Army Medical Corps, was a naturalized American citizen. Among other members of the Canadian Nurse Corps, Mary Catherine Nichols Gunn trained in Ferrisburg, Vermont, and initially worked at Nobel Hospital outside Seattle; Annie Main Gee trained at Minneapolis City Hospital with postgraduate studies at New York Polyclinic; and Eleanor Jane McPhedran trained at New York Hospital

School of Nursing and worked in the area for three years after graduating. In all, the training of Canadian nurses and the nursing services they provided were very much in line with American nursing.

In the case of several prominent British nurses cited throughout the work—Kate Luard, Edith Appleton, Dorothea Crewdson—I am arguably on less certain ground. British nurses—veiled and addressed as "Sister"—cannot strictly speaking play a role in American nursing practice during the Great War. I include them nonetheless for several reasons. The fact is that many British nurses, no less than the Canadians, served abroad for the duration of the war; usually their wartime service extended beyond the Armistice of November 1918 by up to a year. The duration of their wartime experience makes their diaries and letters, taken en masse, more revelatory of treatment-related issues than those of their American colleagues, whose term of service was a year or less. The reflections of Canadian and British nurses on nursing practice on the Western front lend illustrative force to the same battlefield injuries, systemic infections, and psychological traumata encountered by the American nurses.

Shared nursing practices were reinforced by considerable interchange among the allied nurses. Within months of the outbreak of war, American Red Cross (ARC) nurses, all native born and white per ARC requirements, sailed to Europe to lend a hand. On September 12, 1914, the first 126 departed from New York Harbor on a relief ship officially renamed *Red Cross* for the duration of the voyage. A second group of 12 nurses joined three surgeons on a separate vessel destined for Serbia. Other nurse contingents followed over the next several months, all part of the American Red Cross's "Mercy Mission."

Technically ARC nurses were envoys of a neutral nation, and those in the initial group ended up not only in England and France but in Russia, Austro-Hungary, and Germany as well. In the last the ARC worked in concert with the German Red Cross, and American nurses like Caroline Bauer, stationed in Kosel, Germany in 1915, expressed genuine fondness for the "brave and good" German soldiers under her care. For the majority of nurses, however, pre–1917 service in British and French hospitals, despite some initial tensions with British supervisors, reinforced ideological and emotional bonds and introduced American nurses to the realities of combat nursing on the Western front.

Even after America's entry into the war in 1917, American nurses were typically assigned on arrival to British or Canadian hospitals, where they continued their tutelage under senior Canadian and British nursing sisters until returning to their units once their hospitals were ready for them. Allowing for occasional exceptions, the same medicines (sometimes with different names) were administered, the same procedures performed, and the same technologies employed by the nurses of the allied nations. To ignore what the Canadian and British nurses have to say about the same issues of nursing practice encountered by the Americans would enervate the study without leading to any refinement of its thesis.

And so, aided by the testimony of Canadian and British nurses, I am secure in my thesis as it pertains to American nursing and the birth of modern nursing practice. That being said, I leave it to scholars more knowledgeable than I about Canadian and British nursing history to validate, amend, or reject the thesis in relation to their respective nations.

Finally, it bears noting that in a work about nursing practice that draws on the recollections of a cohort of American, Canadian, and British nurses, each nurse is very much her own person with a unique story to tell. The memoirs, letters, and diaries that frame this study provide elements of these stories. In a general way, reactions to the actualities of nursing on the Western front fall along a spectrum of psychological and existential possibilities. At one pole is the affirmation of the combat nursing life provided by Dorothea Crewdson: "I enjoy life here very much indeed. Wonderfully healthy and free." At the opposite pole are the chilling reflections of Mary Borden, for whom "The nurse is no longer a woman. She is dead already, just as I am—really dead, and past resurrection." The gamut of reactions, and the richly idiomatic language through which they were expressed, are woven into this narrative at every turn. I am most concerned, however, with the nurses' transition from one mindset to another, especially the abruptness with which the life-affirming brio of Crewdson gave way to the macabre ruminations of Borden. The happy excitement and prideful sense of participation in the war effort with which American nurses set out for the Front often dissipated shortly after they arrived and saw the human wreckage that would be the locus of their "nursing."

Signposts of personal transformation, which I gather together as epiphanies, represent my point of departure in chapter 1. But in the chapters that follow, these elements of personal biography are subordinate to my focus on nursing practice through a cohort analysis. Fleshing out the individual stories that undergirded such transformations—the chronicles of strong, often overpowering emotions that took nurses to the point of physical and nervous collapse—is the stuff of biography and falls beyond the task I have set myself. It suffices to recall that nurses, no less than the soldiers they cared for, fell victim to what, in the parlance of the war, was termed "shell shock," even though medical and military personnel steadfastly refused to pin this label on them. But most of the time the nurses' descent into the horrific gave rise to adaptive strategies—compartmentalization, dissociation, psychic numbing, black humor—that enabled them to labor on in the service of their soldiers, their "boys."

It is with respect to the nurses' shared ability to bracket their personal stories in the service of a nascent professionalism—a professionalism that segued into a level of autonomous functioning far removed from the world of their training and prewar experience—that they reached their full stature. In so doing, they provide a historical example, deeply moving, of the kind of self-overcoming for which we reserve the term hero.

1

Epiphanies

"Real war at last. Can hardly wait. Here we go!"[1]

It was the all-too-common story of the World War I nurses, the narrative thread that linked the vagaries of their wartime experiences. The war was to be the adventure of a lifetime. The opportunity to serve on the Western front was not to be missed, not by hospital-trained nurses and not by the equally well-trained volunteer Red Cross nurses. For both groups, the call to duty was suffused with the excitement of grand adventure.

Beginning in the spring of 1917, the war abroad was the event of the season, and trained nurses and untrained volunteers rushed to the welcoming embrace of the American Red Cross and the fledging Army Nurse Corps. Julia Stimson, a Vassar graduate who led the St. Louis base hospital unit to Europe in May 1917, was overwhelmed with the honor bestowed on her and the opportunities it promised. "To be in the front ranks in this most dramatic event that ever was staged," she wrote her mother, was "all too much good fortune for any one person like me."[2] Helen Fairchild, an army reserve nurse whose Pennsylvania Hospital Red Cross unit shared space on the SS *St. Paul* with Julia Stimson's St. Louis contingent, wrote her brother and mother in transit: "Our two groups of nurses, the one from St. Louis under Miss Julia C. Stimson and our group from Philadelphia are really excited to be part of this great adventure."[3]

Nurse Fairchild's only problem was seasickness occasioned by a "rocking and rolling" ocean, but no amount of nausea could dampen the sheer exhilaration of the whole thing. A few days later, she wrote her mother of the nurses' memorable send-off at Philadelphia harbor:

9

I must say, it was pretty exciting down at the docks when we left on Saturday. All sizes of boats in the harbor tooted and blew their whistles at us, and people on ferry boats waved and cheered. I know you couldn't be there to see us off and I was thinking of you, but my mind was distracted. How strange everything seemed, but oh how exciting![4]

The fanfare was worlds removed from Fairchild's forebears, the women hospital workers of the American Civil War. They made their own travel plans and journeyed to hospitals at their own expense, often with the disapproval of friends, family, and society at large. In mid-nineteenth-century America, after all, hospitals of any sort remained charitable institutions tainted, the historian Jane Schultz remarks, by "an aura of stigma of sexual impropriety."[5] But this bit of recent history was long forgotten in the mania of 1917. On the deck of the *St. Paul*, Julia Stimson did nothing to calm down the nurses in her charge. Rather, she whipped them up still further. Borrowing language from a letter to her mother, she sounds more like a stellar athlete chosen to represent her nation in the Olympic Games than a nursing administrator headed for the Western front. For Stimson,

to be in the front ranks in this most dramatic event that ever was staged, and to be in the first group of women ever called out for duty with the United States Army, and in the first part of an army ever sent on an expeditionary affair of this sort, is all too much good fortune for any persons like me.[6]

The American nurses who followed Stimson, Fairchild, and others in the fall of 1917 and spring of 1918 were no less welcoming of adventure abroad than the first wave of the preceding summer. Absent any understanding of what lay before them, gaiety abounded, and the trip over could take on the ambience of a holiday cruise. "Heaps of fun … a dandy dance last night … thrilling out today…" are among the diary entries of Ella Mae Bongard, who crossed the Atlantic in October 1917. Born in provincial Ontario but trained and employed in New York City, Bongard wrote the following from somewhere in the North Atlantic on October 9:

Field day sports today, Sack races, potato races, submarine suit races, obstacle, running & eating races. I participated in most of them but have nothing to show for it all but two black knees and a loose tooth all acquired by hitting the deck in the sack & submarine races…. Prizes were distributed after dinner this evening by one of General Scott's aides.[7]

For others it was precisely the anticipation of what lay ahead that made the trip a holiday adventure. They were fearless in the face of mechanized warfare, gangrenous wounds, and poison gas. For 28-year-old Shirley Millard, a Red Cross volunteer nurse from Portland, Oregon, rushed to a field hospital near Soissons in March 1918, the prospect of nursing work at Chateau Gabriel, close to the front, was a dream come true: "It is so exciting and we are all thrilled to have such luck. Real war at last. Can hardly wait. Here we go!"

From Minnesotan Grace Anderson, a reserve nurse and nurse-anesthetist who embarked from New York Harbor in July 1918, came a bold and joyful avowal: "I haven't the least fear or worry in the world. Am ready for anything."[8] For Millard, Anderson, Bongard and countless others, serving in a base hospital or, more exciting still, in a field hospital or casualty clearing station (CCS) only a few miles from the front, was to be invited to the Grand Cotillion. Volunteer Red Cross and regular army nurses alike were well-bred young women of substance—typically upper-middle or upper-class and college-educated substance. So yes, they were adventuresome and patriotic and given over to a sense of duty shaped by literary culture, not battlefield experience. So they experienced happiness on receiving the call; they would do themselves proud and make their families proud.

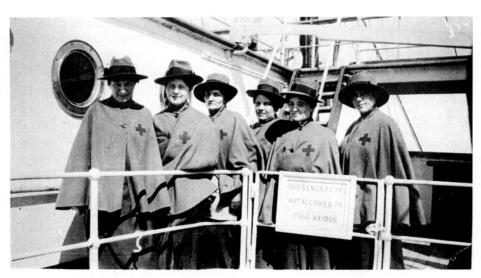

A group of American Red Cross nurses en route to France in 1918. Some 9,000 Red Cross nurses enlisted in the Army and saw active duty abroad during World War I (Library of Congress).

How are we to understand their excitement about battlefield nursing in the modern, mechanistic world of 1917? Did they not understand they would be treating wounds so massive that they could leave imperceptible the humanness of the mutilated object before them? Or treating infections so severe that they led to anguished deaths in a matter of minutes or hours or days? Had they not read popular accounts or viewed images of soldiers in the agonized aftermath of poison gas attacks? Could they not imagine soldiers whose suffering was so intense and unremitting that it could drive soldier and nurse alike to the point of breakdown, even madness?

And that is precisely the point: What awaited the American nurses after their shipboard adventures lay far outside anything they *could* have imagined. In place of newspaper accounts about the nature and extent of the suffering and dying on the front—the catastrophic wounds inflicted by large artillery, shrapnel, and poison gas—they, like virtually all Americans, clung to the stories of their elders. The young nurses, no less than the young men who, beginning on June 5, 1917, flooded U.S. army recruitment centers, grew up in the shadow of the Civil War, when surviving veterans like Oliver Wendell Holmes, Jr.—the generation of their grandfathers—along with countless boys who, like Theodore Roosevelt and Woodrow Wilson, grew up in their worshipful shadow—the generation of their fathers—persisted in cloaking war in what David Kennedy terms a "spirit of chivalric gallantry."

For the generation of 1917, as for the two generations that preceded it, war was the event of a lifetime, "a liberating release from the stultifying conventions of civilized society."[9] The same had been true, perhaps even more so, for the British nurses who steamed to South Africa in the fall of 1899 when Britain, for the second time in two decades, went to war against the Boer republics. For these nurses, devotion to the empire and its imperial mission barely masked excitement at escaping Victorian constraints on social behavior, visiting an exotic part of the world sans chaperones, and collecting welcome pay (and souvenirs) for their patriotic service abroad. Unlike the Americans of 1917, however, the nurses of the Second Anglo-Boer War did not enter an expansive three-year war zone with an intricate network of casualty clearing stations (CCSs), field hospitals, stationary hospitals, base hospitals, and general hospitals, all up and running and staffed by seasoned European, Canadian, and Australian nurses.

Compared to the American nurses of 1917, the British nurses of 1899 rather tiptoed into wartime nursing. Limited at first to base hospitals a distance from what passed for the front, they encountered no seriously wounded troops on arrival and contented themselves with the less onerous challenge of the poor sanitation and overcrowding of the military camps.[10] This was entirely to the liking of the 100 members of the Army Medical Service (AMS), Supervising Sisters whose work in British military hospitals was limited to monitoring the orderlies who provided all hands-on care, taking temperatures and administering medications and stimulants distributed by the Sisters. The larger contingent of 800 British and colonial civilian nurses who filled the ranks were resented by the AMS regulars, not only because they only enlisted for the duration of the war, but because, as caregivers, they were better trained and more activist as providers, criticizing the army orderlies and often preempting them at patients' bedsides.[11]

It was worse still for the American nurses who steamed to Cuba and the Philippines to serve in the four-month Spanish-American War of 1898. They encountered living conditions no less primitive than the British, but lacked nursing supplies that were desperately needed at the time of arrival. For the American nurses of 1898, there was no period of acclimation and little sense of patriotic adventure in the stifling wards of typhoid, malaria, yellow fever, and dysenteric patients who awaited them. Their participation in America's first imperialist foray had not been anticipated by Surgeon General George Sternberg, who, with the blessing of Congress, signed up female nurses under contract ("contract nurses") only when confronted with the typhoid epidemic raging through federal training camps in the South. In May, seven percent of the troops had taken ill, and by August it had climbed to 28 percent, with 53,705 camp hospital admissions and 776 deaths in an army of 190,347. The nurses who were sent contracts for army service were prescreened and approved by a committee of members of the Daughters of the American Revolution (DAR) headed by Dr. Anita Newcomb McGee, a practicing physician from Washington, D.C., and DAR vice president. They began arriving in May and, to the surprise of surgeons and the War Department alike, provided exemplary service under the most onerous circumstances. At Georgia's Camp Thomas, the major staging area for the war, they worked 14-hour shifts caring for typhoid victims, many delirious, who required nourishment every two hours, several ice baths daily, additional care of the skin and mouth, and physical therapy.[12]

Having proven themselves up to the rigors (and filth) of military camp life, some of the nurses followed the troops to Cuba, where typhoid fever and yellow fever had sapped the army's fighting strength, and then to Puerto Rico and the Philippines. One such nurse, Amy Wingreen, a Chicagoan trained at Cook County Hospital, was transferred to a yellow fever ward with 72 patients shortly after her arrival. On returning to the United States, she grimly reflected: "We had no floors in the sick tents or in any tents, a limited supply of remedies, no ice scarcely, no proper amount of food and clothing, and rains several times a day soaking many of the sick ones."[13]

It was different for the Americans of 1917. No less than the male enlistees, the U.S. Army Corps nurses heading to Europe imbibed a view of war not merely as grand adventure, but as character-building in beneficent Christian ways. Indeed, their service to the nation was put to them as an absolute good that carried a divine message. This last came from Justice Holmes, addressing Harvard's graduating class of 1895.[14] More than two decades later, when America finally entered the Great War, the medieval view of war as a Christian struggle both elevated and elevating—a struggle in which the wounds of the battlefield would be ennobling and heroically borne—saturated American newspapers, popular magazines, novels, and movies. The nurses' bracing sense of adventure was shaped by a war that began almost three years earlier and, notwithstanding the nation's formal neutrality, featured allies and enemies from the outset. So the liberation of American nurses was less about social and sexual mores than a rare and golden opportunity to do good for themselves, their country, and all mankind. How could they refuse service? Had not *The Biblical World* intoned in its March 1917 issue that

> a war in the defense of the spiritual precipitate of civilization is justifiable; in the last resort it is a duty. For it is a less evil than the loss of spiritual achievements. War to preserve ideals is better than moral anarchy, however scientific or euphemized.[15]

The Christianizing of the war hardly awaited America's belated entry in April 1917. It was integral to Americans' appreciation of the war throughout the extended period of political neutrality. No sooner had a German U-20 type U-boat torpedoed the British ocean liner *Lusitania* on May 7, 1915, than the *North American Review* lauded the Allies as the champions "of liberty, of humanity, of Christianity" against "the Satanic powers of Germany."[16] By the time America entered the war on April 6, 1917, the country's progressive Christian leaders, key shapers of public opinion, had abandoned pacifism for a crusading interventionism in which entry into the war was a Christian imperative. In making the world safe for democracy, it would usher in the dream of the ancient Christians: an everlasting kingdom of peace, justice, and righteousness.[17]

The Christianizing of the war in Europe came easily to America's young men who were called on to fight it. Theirs was the world of muscular Christianity, of Christ as militant warrior savagely battling forces of evil. Well before 1914, the masculinization of Christ's message fed the growth of youth groups, both inside and outside mainstream Protestant churches, seeking to cultivate in young people a strenuous, aggressive Christian faith. The warrior ideal was everywhere; it gained expression in the histrionic sermons of the wildly popular evangelist Billy Sunday and popular books such as Carl Delos Case's *The Masculine in Religion* (1906), Jason Pierce's *The Masculine Power of Christ* (1912), and especially Warren Conant's *The Virility of Christ*, published in 1904 and reissued in 1915.[18] It stood to reason that when the call to arms came in April 1917, American troops were primed to view it as what Jonathan Ebel terms "an arena in which faith could be lived out, tested, and animated." As they boarded transport ships, sometimes sharing space with the nurses who would care for them, they viewed what lay ahead less as a conventional war between nations than a redemptive mission in which personal meanings were enveloped in a cosmic struggle between good and evil, a struggle in which "the fate of civilized Christian humanity hung in the balance."[19]

The nurses who headed to Europe in 1917 and 1918 were hardly immune to the message of muscular Christianity. As women, they were a decisive step removed from the ideal of the male warrior but no less excited and, given the rightness of their cause, no less fearless. They were children of their time, their childhoods shaped by the same cultural myths and messianic gloss as those of the men. And they too were among the elect: They were chosen to participate in what Princeton University President John Grier Hibben termed the chastening and purifying effect of armed conflict. How not to feel proud about joining in a war that promised, in the words of the contemporary novelist Robert Herrick, a "resurrection of nobility."[20]

Only a handful of these nurses had served in the Spanish-American War,[21] that four-month exercise in rank imperialism that never seeped into the popular imagination and was eclipsed altogether by the events of 1914. Nor were the nurses who set sail for Europe in 1917 and 1918 the daughters of working-class or petit-bourgeois fathers. They were white, well-bred, and well-read. No less than their male counterparts, whether enlisted men or officers, they were among the elite, "the nation's most carefully cultivated youths, the privileged recipients of the finest education, steeped in the values of the genteel tradition, who most believe the archaic doctrines about war's noble and heroic possibilities."[22] "Gee," wrote Helen Fairchild from the deck of the *St. Paul*, "half of our enlisted men are millionaires or millionaire's sons, and as for the doctors, well, Philadelphia does not have men any finer..."[23] The nurses were no less fine. They were happily self-satisfied, often jubilant, at getting on board, physically, mentally, spiritually, and joining a struggle that promised to revitalize American cultural self-awareness, reaffirm its moral idealism, and, if the liberal clergy were to be believed, usher in a new Christian world order.

The U-boat infested waters into which the nurses steamed failed to dim the overall gaiety of the whole thing. At the very time Helen Fairchild boarded the *St. Paul*, reports arrived of an American transport already at sea that had spotted a submarine; on the same ship a short time later, nurses on deck watched a torpedo approach—and miss—their ship. But Fairchild's glowing sense of the adventure before her was undiminished. Isabel Anderson was a Boston socialist and Red Cross volunteer, and when her transport ship, the French-built *Espagne*, reached the danger zone outside the British Isles, Anderson and her friends assembled on deck in "frog-like rubber life-saving suits" in front of the life boats. But they were no more fazed by hazardous seas than Fairchild: "Six of us women slept side by side in a corner on deck, with our passports and money upon us and our life-belts beside us—it was very warm below—and we told stories and giggled like school girls. Even if the bed was hard, it was fun to watch people prowling round in the darkness." For Emma Elizabeth Weaver, a Red Cross nurse who joined the University of Penn-

sylvania Unit in mid–February 1918 and embarked for France the following May on the gigantic transport *Leviathan*, there was less excitement than a love of the sea so deep and abiding that she wished the
voyage would never end. No more than for Fairchild or Anderson
did imminent disaster temper her pleasure at being at sea. "I love the
motion of the boat, to be rocked to sleep at night," she wrote in her
journal, and then, without pause, added: "We missed a torpedo by
five seconds."[24]

• • •

After enduring seasickness, morning calisthenics, and lifeboat
drills, the nurses reached their arrival ports of Liverpool and Brest,
and the celebration began all over again. They were wined, dined,
paraded—feted by royalty in every manner befitting America's heroic
liberators. And then, after partying and shopping and socializing,
they finally crossed the English Channel and reached their military
destinations. And within a matter of hours, or days, or, if they were
lucky, a week or two, their exhilaration at being invited to a Patriotic
Ball quickly gave way to stunned amazement at the actual "work"
before them. Typically assigned to British or French field hospitals
while their own were being built, the American nurses soon encountered wounds that were literally unimaginable to them, and then in
the fevered atmosphere of post-battle rushes, became wrenchingly
imaginable, indeed omnipresent. Quickly they grew familiar with the
horrid stench of gas gangrene, which crackled beneath the surface
of infected body parts and almost always presaged quick death. Under
the mentoring of senior nurses, the young Americans learned how
to prep patients for surgery, including cases in which "there are only
pieces of men left." And yet, left with no choice, they quickly made
their peace with the stumps of severed limbs and concavities of missing stomachs, faces, and eyes, and began to help clean, irrigate, and
dress what remained, before and after surgery, if surgery could even
be attempted.

Like the European and Canadian nurses who preceded them and
alongside whom they worked, the Americans learned, with few
exceptions, to remain unflinching in the face of each soldier who
arrived at the casualty clearing station "unrecognizable as a human
being." And they learned to remain composed before soldiers as
young as fourteen—"children" or "little boys" or "poor youngsters"

or "infants,"[25] they would say—who arrived caked in mud and blood and covered with lice. Multiple wounds abounded. A soldier is wounded in seven places and a hip was blown off; another arrived with both legs and his left arm broken and his face "pitifully cut up."[26] An anonymous nurse working in a Belgian field hospital tells her diary of a soldier who

> came in with his arm broken in several places and bleeding; in his abdomen were two large wounds which had pierced the intestine in several places. He also had a great wound in the back which had smashed up one kidney. At first he was too collapsed to operate upon.[27]

Three wounds, five wounds, seven wounds, nine wounds, eleven wounds.[28] There is no respite from the multiply wounded. Here "a poor youngster with both legs broken, both arms wounded, one eye shot out and the other badly damaged"; there a "poor lad" who "had both eyes shot through and there they were, all smashed and mixed up with the eyelashes. He was quite calm, and very tired. He said, 'Shall I need an operation? I can't see anything.'" Within a week of her arrival at a French field hospital, Shirley Millard, who hailed from Portland, Oregon, wrote of bathing a patient's "great hip cavity where a leg once was." While she did so, "a long row of others, their eyes fastened upon me, await their turn." And then she offered the kind of litany that countless others offered: "Gashes from bayonets. Flesh torn by shrapnel. Faces half shot away. Eyes seared by gas; one here with no eyes at all. I can see down into the back of his head." Another soldier with gangrenous wounds oozing everywhere quickly morphs into a "mass of very putrid rottenness before the nurse's eyes and long before he dies." Such was the experience of Edith Appleton, who continued: "The smell was so very terrible I had to move him right away from everyone, and all one could do was dress and redress. Happily I don't think he could smell it himself but I have never breathed a worse poison."[29]

All too soon after arrival, the cheery young American nurses beheld the fearless young soldiers—or remnants thereof—who came to them in funeral processions of ambulances. And they saw that the fearless young men had become "wretched, restless beings." This is Shirley Millard, whose diary entry continues: "The crowded, twisted bodies, the screams and groans, made one think of the old engraving in Dante's *Inferno*. More came, and still more." For Helen

Boylston, who trained at Massachusetts General Hospital and travelled to Europe with the Harvard Medical Unit, a "rush" during the final German offensive of late August 1918 brought 1,100 wounded to her base hospital in 24 hours, with three operating teams performing some 90 emergency operations that night and the nights to follow. The operating room nurse, she recalled, "walked up and down between the tables with a bottle of aromatic spirits of ammonia in one hand and a bottle of brandy in the other, ready to pounce on the next person who wilted." At Beatrice Hopkinson's CCS 47, just outside Amiens, the situation was more dire still. During the March rush many thousands of patients passed through the doors in only a few days and kept seven operating tables working day and night.[30]

• • •

And so the narratives captured in the diaries, journals, and memoirs of the American nurses, no less than those of the British and Canadian nurses, turned a corner and peered into blackness. For many, the fight for God's kingdom on earth mutated into something grotesque, much closer to a Hell on Earth. The nurses experienced epiphanies of radical disillusionment, their sense of mission jeopardized and their values destabilized. Eventually, their lives were reshaped—or was it deformed?—through the actualities of nursing on the Western front, which included both an inability to nurse back to life many of the war wounded, and an ability to nurse back to life many who returned to the front to be reinjured and killed. This was especially true of young civilian nurses who enlisted for the war, many little older than the combatants, who in no time at all became war-weary and war-wise in ways that choked off the exhilaration that carried them to European shores.

The nurses' epiphanies are shorn of Latinate layers of ecclesiastical meaning. They connect rather with the ancient Greek *epiphaneia*, which denotes a manifestation, a bringing to light, a sudden coming into view. For the nurses the coming into view was tantamount to a sudden, often dramatic, coming into focus of the reality of their participation in a panorama of suffering, mutilation, dismemberment, blindness, and death—and the excoriated dehumanized landscape that all the patriotic killing left behind.

The nurses' epiphanies arise from the shared context of battle-field nursing, but they still evince variety. They can arise from the psychological equivalent of a slow pressure cooker, where a vague sense of dis-ease, of ineffectiveness, builds up over time and gives way to intermittently conscious feelings of futility. Moments of futility increase, until finally exploding into a crystal-clear revelation about war and the profound limitations of nursing care as an anodyne for the pain, suffering, and dying that not only occur during war but constitute war. At other times epiphanies have no apparent buildup; they erupt full-blown out of an existential nowhere.

Among the nurses of World War I, there are epiphanies of impotence, epiphanies about what the nursing self can and cannot do. Such epiphanies can be more or less delimited, dealing, for example, with suitability for the nursing vocation. Thus the Canadian nurse Agnes Warner: "I think I shall have to find a new job when war is over, for I don't think I shall ever do any more nursing." Other nurses cannot think beyond the war. Instead, they dig in deeper and fashion a gendered sense of obligation to nurse on, and thereby contain the horror seeping into their personal nursing space. Thus the Boston Brahmin Nora Saltonstall, a Red Cross nurse who became a member of a mobile hospital unit, an *Autochir*, that followed combatants throughout northern France: "I have seen enough wounded and dying to hate the war, but I believe in having women to nurse them even if the women are in danger, because the moral effect on the men is beyond belief."[31]

But the moral uplift of female nursing on the wounded does not always valorize the nurses themselves. Some experience epiphanies of despair with the realization that, by enabling soldiers to recover from their wounds and infections and return to the Front, they paradoxically become instruments of death:

> I never realized the war so much until this last convoy. I wonder if it's ever going to end. It seems so senseless to keep sending well men up to the line to be shot to pieces.[32]
> Sometimes I almost dread seeing them recover so rapidly, as it only meant that they had to return to the horror of it all again.[33]

There are surprising, even unsettling, epiphanies of humanization that occur when nurses care for enemy prisoners. At *L'Hôpital Jacobean*, Alice Isaacson, an American-trained Canadian nurse assigned to the French Army, beholds a ward run by an American nurse. There, the permanently crippled were taught various trades best adapted to their particular disability. And the strange thing about this hive of industry is that German prisoners were teaching these trades to the victims of their shell fire: "And they appear to be on the best of terms, working happily together. The Germans are adept workmen specially chosen for this work."[34]

For Canadian Kate Wilson, working at a British casualty clearing station only five miles behind the Somme front, the epiphany of humanization is more brutally direct: "One look at his terrified face and he was no longer a hated Hun, just a small wounded boy without a friend on any side. What hurt the most was the fact that he was frightened of me."[35]

Many epiphanies are triggered by intimate contact with one, perhaps one too many, severely injured dying soldiers. Others have nothing at all to do with soldiers. Consider Emma Elizabeth Weaver, whose idyllic sea voyage of April 1918 was followed by wartime service at Base Hospital 20 and then an eight-month stint with the Army of Occupation in Coblenz, Germany. In a journal entry from January 1919, she records a train ride from Paris to Metz when a casual glance out the window led to an especially painful, poignant moment: "Really, I don't know when anything ever made me feel so badly as the sight of a civilian cemetery we passed."[36]

Other epiphanic moments involve the nonhuman victims of war. These epiphanies are deeply affecting because the process of humanizing reaches out from the humans who make war to the innocent animals who suffer from it. It is no longer the enemy in the person of a frightened boy soldier who jolts a nurse into renewed appreciation of shared humanity. Rather it comes from witnessing the senseless sacrifice of the only true innocents on the battlefield, on whose backs the cavalry leads the charge. During the American Civil War, the Union nurse Sophronia Bucklin, surveying the battlefield wreckage in northern Virginia in 1863, records just such an epiphanic moment:

> I think the most pitiful sight I ever beheld was that of one of these skeleton creatures lying in the stagnant water of a little brook, whither he had doubtless gone to drink, and falling in was too exhausted to rise. As we neared him the instinct of human presence seemed to nerve him with some little vigor, for he raised his head and neighed imploringly—the glassy eyes even then glaring with death. We could not help the dying creature, and for days the scene haunted my mind.[37]

And now in the winter of 1916, American-born Lucille Ross Jones has another such epiphany, this one occasioned by the slaughter of wounded horses whose meat, she well knows, will feed tubercular patients. "It just wrings my heart," she writes, "when I pass by the place and see a poor old horse waiting for his turn to be killed. But I suppose it is better than letting him live and suffer. What a lot of cruelty there is in this war!"[38]

All too often dehumanized wartime slaughter bursts the bounds of pity and gives way to epiphanies of disgust, which mingled with infinite sadness. Blindness is catastrophic disability, and encountering soldiers blinded on the battlefield frequently provokes an epiphany. Here once more is Alice Isaacson as she watches a wounded Frenchman, a *poilus*, help a blinded comrade to the altar to seek the consolation of religion. Isaacson finds the scene "pathetic" and angrily writes: "Europe and Canada are leaving this awful burden of blindness, because of the selfish ambition of a few men in high places."[39] Among soldiers exposed to poison gas, first used by the Germans during the second battle of Ypres in the spring of 1915, blindness, sometimes temporary, becomes endemic. Helen Dore Boylston presents an indelible image that affected her for life and affects us still:

> There were strings of from eight to twenty blind boys filing up the road, clinging tightly and pitifully to each other's hands, and led by some bedraggled limping youngster who could still see.... I wonder if I'll ever be able to look at marching men anywhere again without seeing those blinded boys, with five and six wound stripes on their sleeves, struggling painfully along the road.[40]

And then, finally, there are epiphanies of more general philosophical import. Call them epiphanies of skeptical enlightenment, bitterly toned and angrily resigned. For nurses such as Helen Boylston, Mary Borden, and Ellen LaMotte, war brought them to the threshold of their own nonnegotiable no-man's land, a psychic zone where numbing preempts epiphanies of humanization. The nurse, writes Mary Borden in *The Forbidden Zone*,

> is no longer a woman. She is dead already, just as I am—really dead, past resurrection. Her heart is dead. She killed it. She couldn't bear to feel it jumping in her side when Life, the sick animal, choked and rattled in her arms. Her ears are deaf; she deafened them. She could not bear to hear Life crying and mewing. She is blind so that she cannot see the torn parts of men she must handle. Blind, deaf, dead—she is strong, efficient, fit to consort with gods and demons—a machine inhabited by the ghost of a woman—soulless, past redeeming, just as I am—just as I will be.[41]

For Borden, it is affective de-humanization, what a later generation of military psychiatrists would term psychic numbing, that enables nurses to bear up, even as they were ground down, their patriotic values pulverized to dust. Comprehending trench warfare in bodily perspective, they become freighted with the pointlessness of the horror, which in tented clearing stations and hospitals, came down to multitudes of mutilated, infection-saturated, and lifeless young bodies. Helen Boylston felt it too, and believed the sheer stupidity of the whole business supplanted any possibility of the tragic.

> Today a ditch is full of Germans, and tomorrow it is full of Englishmen. Neither side really wants the silly muddy ditch, yet they kill each other persistently, wearily, ferociously, patiently, in order to gain possession of it. And whoever wins, it has won—nothing.[42]

Nurse-philosophers ponder the paradox of pain—the impossibility of knowing its nature in another along with the inability to nurse without imagining it. Over time, they acquire the capacity to feel shame— shame in their own strength, as in their ability to stand firm and straight alongside a bedside "whose coverings are flung here and there by the quivering nerves beneath it." They empathize with shell-shocked patients who, having endured the prospect of "glorious death" under the guns, were sent home "to face death in another form. Not glorious, shameful." And finally there is the shame, thinly veiled, attendant to witnessing the unremitting pain of the dying. "No philosophy," reflects Enid Bagnold, "helps the pain of death. It is pity, pity, pity, that I feel, and sometimes a sort of shame that I am here to write at all."[43]

As hostilities drew to a close in the fall of 1918, the most expansive reflections of all, the alterations of life philosophy that grew out of wartime nursing, were set down. At war's end, Helen Boylston is herself a patient at Britain's General Hospital No. 22 in Camiers, France. Flat on her back, feverish and "as yellow as a cow-lily," she records these thoughts in a diary entry of November 19, 1918, eight days after the Armistice ending hostilities has been signed:

> The war has done strange things to me. It has given me a lot and taken away a lot. It has taught me that nothing matters, really. That people do not matter, and things do not matter, and laces do not matter, except for a minute. And the minute is always now.[44]

For Oregonian Shirley Millard, Armistice Day and the immediate dismissal of her unit of Red Cross nurses marked her epiphany:

Only then did the enormous crime of the whole thing begin to come home to me. All very well to celebrate, I thought, but what about Charley? All the Charlies? What about Donnelly, Goldfarb, Wendel, Auerbach? And René? And the hundreds, thousands of others.[45]

The enormity of the crime and the absurd reasoning that justified it coalesced in the wartime essays of the two most gifted essayists of the postwar era, Mary Borden and Ellen LaMotte. Borden was a Chicago heiress and Vassar graduate whose inherited wealth enabled her to staff and equip her own front-line mobile hospital for the French army. La Motte was a graduate of Johns Hopkins Training School, an expert tubercular nurse in Baltimore, and a budding social reformer and writer. Together, they articulate a vision of war that transcends issues of suffering, loss, and grief. Both nurses expatiate less on the suffering and loss of life than on war's sheer grotesquerie. A recurrent theme for both is the impossibility of the good death in war, where the very effort to "restore" bodies and minds that are shattered, literally and figuratively, becomes oxymoronic. War, both writers insist, can only be situated in an alternate universe where any claim to morality is, from the standpoint of ordinary human life, self-willed delusion. In this universe cavalier surgeons function as automatons, and even their life-saving interventions are specious, since the lives they save, more often than not, are no longer human lives, psychologically or physically. In this parody of ordinary existence, the moral fabric of being has not merely been rent but twisted into a hideous inversion of itself, one in which death withheld, paradoxically, is the ultimate act of inhumanity.[46]

What makes the nurses of World War I gallants is that they were able to bracket the encroaching horror, with its undercurrents of rage, depression, and numbing—and simply care for their patients. They were able to function as nurses in a nurses' hell. Military directives pushed them to an even lower circle of a caregiver's *Inferno*, since their primary task, they were told again and again, was to get injured troops back to the front as soon as possible. The nurses were to fix up serviceable (and hence service-able) soldiers so that they could be reused at least one more time before breakdown, physical or mental, precluded further remedial servicing and the soldier's obligation to serve further.

But the nurses knew better and unfailingly did better. Nursing practice, it turns out, had its own moral imperative, in the light of which military directives could be downplayed, often cast to the wind. As the nursing historian Christine Hallett observes, the emotional containment nurses provided for suffering and needy soldiers did not, indeed *could* not, preclude caring.[47] In chapters to follow, I hope to explore further the remarkable elements of this caring, which blurred the boundary between comfort care and healing and took nursing practice into the realm of emergency medicine, management of infectious disease, surgery, orthopedics, and psychotherapy. It is as agents of caregiving that trespassed the boundaries of nursing and medicine in the patient's interest that the nurses of World War I rose to the status of gallants. Flying in the face of military priorities, surgical fatalism, and their own crises of professional and moral self-worth, they bravely pursued cure where cure was impossible. This is the "cure" that is true to the word's etymology, the Latin *curare*, which is a *taking care of* that privileges the patient's welfare above all else.

• • •

"They nursed on." What does this mean, and what does it mean especially from one war to another? Military and nursing historians—with several noteworthy exceptions[48]—tend to finesse this very basic historical question. For nurses in one or another war, they provide richly informative accounts of the military environments in which nurses served, dwelling especially on the exigent circumstances, on and off the battlefield, in which they often find themselves. Topical studies of military nurses tell about the family circumstances and upbringing of nurses: their training, prewar work, and the circumstances that led to wartime service. Where sources permit, they write of their relationship to medical and military authorities; their interactions with patients; their fear and courage while under attack; the institutional arrangements that structured their lives; and the social (and occasionally romantic) lives they managed to lead outside these structures.

But as to the actual nursing activities of wartime nurses, much less is said. Many writers, nurses among them, want to view "nursing" almost metaphysically as a kind of caregiving that in certain respects is timeless. Nursing, *all* nursing, eases suffering and promotes healing, at least according to the prevalent theories that guide nursing and medical care alike. Nurses also promoted comfort by attending to metabolic and regulatory needs. There is nothing profound about such nursing, whatever the historical period in which a particular war occurs. Nurses provide hungry patients with food and thirsty patients with drink. They bring blankets to patients who are cold and ice and cold compresses to patients who are hot. They aid patients in expelling waste and keep them as clean and dry as circumstances permit. They administer medication—whatever that means at a particular point in medical history—often but not always as directed by doctors. They summon doctors when warning signs suggest a patient is not responding to treatment or suffering unduly or dying. And, as patient advocates, nurses question doctors' judgment with respect to any number of practices. During the Civil War, for example, a nurse might question a doctor about the amount of morphine he was ordering for his patients.[49]

What I have described is the maternal vision of nursing promulgated by Florence Nightingale after her experience in the Crimean War of 1853–1856. This vision, famously set forth in her *Notes on Nursing: What Nursing Is, What Nursing Is Not* (1859),[50] guided the generally untrained female hospital workers who nursed wounded Union and Confederate troops in the tented field hospitals and cavernous general hospitals of the Civil War. These women, whose nursing bona fides were simply a caring disposition, maternal or otherwise, were embraced by wounded soldiers but viewed with skeptical dislike by surgeons and military officials, especially in the South.

Civil War nurses too nursed on, but "nursing on" meant something quite different for them than for the nurses of World War I. It meant persisting as patient advocates in the inhospitably all-male hospital environments. This meant wresting shipments of food and clothing sent to patients from corrupt quartermasters and military surgeons and redirecting them to the patients for whom they were intended. It meant reporting instances of theft and the physical abuse of patients to authorities, first within the hospital and then, if necessary, outside it. It meant providing religious consolation to the dying and ensuring them of the good life to follow. And it meant touching patients physically and emotionally—holding their hands, listening to their stories, writing their letters home, and promising to write their families after they died.

Certainly Civil War nurses assigned to military units did their share of bandaging, on and off the battlefield. "Equipped for labor with a box of bandages, a box of lint, adhesive plaster, sponge, shears, and chloroform," they ventured onto battlefields immediately after major battles, walking among hundreds, often thousands, of wounded troops wracked with pain and thirst, frequently delirious, often dying agonizing deaths. There they began what the Union nurse Sophronia Bucklin termed their "labor of mercy."[51] Back in the field hospitals, Bucklin and others continued to nurse in the intimate, unladylike manner demanded by circumstance. With hands that "had ceased to tremble when hundreds of worms feasted upon the rank battle-wounds," Bucklin removed, in one memorable instance, "a full pint of dead worms" from a soldier's side, after which she "thoroughly washed out the wound, and filled it with soft lint, wet in cold water, then bandaged him about the waist."[52] Applying cold compresses to infected wounds emanating "fever heat" or vigorously rubbing the extremities of soldiers with severe neuralgic pain—these tasks too fell to nurses. And nurses always took the lead in preparing and applying mustard plasters (i.e., poultices), that mainstay of antebellum remedies for respiratory illness and rheumatic pain.[53]

This was Civil War nursing par excellence. But first and foremost, Civil War nursing was about food, water, and dying. For genteel Southern hospital workers such as Ada Bacot, nursing was a matter of overseeing food preparation, especially the special diets ordered by doctors for particular patients. Bacot, be it noted, occasionally filled special needs on her own, sending syrup to a patient with a wretched cough, for example.[54] For nurses such as Bucklin, the food narrative sometimes veered to desperation. In the battlefields of northern Virginia in the fall of 1863, she depicts the aftermath of battle as a grueling contest between starvation and sustenance for nurses and the wounded alike. Her own hunger intermittently felled her, to the point that, on several occasions, she was unable to take any nourishment except tea for days at a time. Battlefield nursing, beyond bandaging those who could be bandaged, meant securing something, indeed anything, to eat in order to be able to nurse on, the "anything" meaning a bit of pork, sometimes uncooked, moldy hardtack, and worm-infested bread. With such dubious fortification, Bucklin nursed on, which meant securing the same such rations for the starving wounded.

And the starving wounded looked to their nurses for just such sustenance. "One of my former patients," writes Bucklin, "learning that I was on the field, came a mile and a half on crutches to beg of me for something to eat." At which point she ran over to the tent of a kindly sanitary commission worker, who bestowed on her a feast of baked pork and beans and, *mirabile dictu*, a dried apple pie. "Hastening back," she concludes, "I sat it on a corner of the table, and bade him eat."[55]

For other battlefield nurses of the Civil War, the nutritional obligation was given quantitative measure. When Harriet Eaton encountered 30 starving soldier compatriots from her native Maine in a Division Hospital during the battle of Fredericksburg, she stayed with them the afternoon, making "whiskey punch and provided crackers, butter, and marmalade for all the Maine men." Two days later, she allowed herself a rare admission: "Oh! I am so tired, I wonder how many messes of gruel and punch I have made to day [sic]." But for Eaton the quantities and the exhaustion only increase in the days ahead: "four quarts of gruel, four gallons of chicken broth, and as much hot broma [light cocoa] with crackers spread with marmalade" on one day; a full 16 gallons of chicken broth on the next.[56]

And then, ricocheting from the starving collective to the gravely wounded individual, control of food was a marker of nursing authority. Serving as ward matron at Fort Schuyler Hospital on Long Island Sound in the fall of 1862, Emily Parsons took exclusive charge of a seriously ill soldier who had just undergone a reamputation of his arm. Following the surgeon's departure, she "allowed no one else to touch his bed or his food." More impressively still, during the surgeon's subsequent visits he "sometimes pours out his porter, but it is handed me to give."[57] Locating food, selecting food, preparing food, supervising others preparing food, feeding the seriously wounded— these things were not epiphenomenal to nursing service during the Civil War; they were of its essence.

Thirty-five years later, Anita McGee, whose vision of professional nursing made little room for food-related comfort care, did not end her service to the nation by overseeing the selection of contract nurses for the Spanish-American War. Rather, she remained in command and sought to mold army nurses into a corps of professionals for whom expertise supplanted the Nightingalean view of nurses as all-purpose caregivers whose maternalism embraced whatever tasks, menial or otherwise, they were assigned. McGee's organizational success story is well known. We know that her efforts impressed the army brass and War Department sufficiently to have her appointed Acting Assistant Surgeon on August 29, 1898, and that the work of American nurses serving under her dispelled any remaining doubts about the need for a contingent of trained female nurses in wartime. Most notably, it led to the Army Reorganization Act of 1901, drafted by McGee herself, which in turn established the U.S. Army Nurse Corps as a part of the regular Army.

Nor did McGee's crusade for nurse professionalism end with the Spanish-American War. Army nurses imbued with her professionalizing zeal stayed on in Cuba, Puerto Rico, and the Philippines, and fanned out to Hawaii and even China in the following several years. In April 1904, after war broke out between Japan and Russia, McGee herself selected nine Spanish-American War nurses to accompany her to Japan, where, under the aegis of the Japanese Red Cross Society, they set up shop in the army reserve hospital in Hiroshima, a massive base hospital of 14,000 beds, there to help Japanese nurses cope with returning wounded from Manchuria. Appointed Superintendent of Nursing at the hospital, McGee continued as a professionalizing missionary, persuading Japan's medical and military brass that Japanese nurses would better serve the nation and the nation's wounded if they were relieved of housekeeping chores and allowed to develop a level of expertise commensurate with that of their American brethren. Judging from her subsequent report to the Japanese Red Cross Society, McGee enjoyed considerable success, at least insofar as she and her nine colleagues were readily accepted as models of what we would term "best nursing practice" by the Japanese.[58] What kind of actual nursing McGee's cohort was permitted to do is less clear, and journalistic accounts of their status were less flattering.[59]

And yet, the success of McGee and her nursing corps abroad leaves unanswered the same question that arises in the aftermath of her success in the Spanish-American War. To wit, what exactly were the professional skills that graduate nurses brought to bear on wounded American soldiers in 1898 and Japanese soldiers in 1904? On this the literature tells little. The Spanish-American War was less a war of bullet wounds than of rampant infectious disease, especially typhoid fever and yellow fever. What skills were brought to bear in nursing infected soldiers that were not available to untrained volunteer nurses? Any responsible person, after all, can bring a typhoid patient nourishment at regular intervals, administer ice baths, and provide basic skin care.

Clearly, the female nurses' knowledge of bacteriology and the nature of disease transmission set them apart from untrained soldiers assigned to the army's hospital corps to perform nursing duty. A visit to typhoid-ridden Camp Thomas in August 1898 found a camp where male "nurses" who were "worthless men ... ignorant, filthy men," drawn from regiments that found them unfit to serve in battle. On their arrival at the camp in the fall of 1898, two graduate nurses from New York City reported conditions so unsanitary and primitive that it was only by the grace of God that any survivors remained.[60]

It was the training of the graduate nurses that enabled them to stabilize the situation and begin to turn it around. Major breakthroughs in the understanding and treatment of typhoid were occurring around the very time they arrived—the first typhoid vaccine had been successfully given to 14,000 British troops during the Boer War and, on the conclusion of the Spanish-American War, the Typhoid Commission appointed by President McKinley determined that typhoid had been transmitted in the camps by human contact.[61] But the former fact was unknown to them and the latter lay in the future. McGee's nurses had no special knowledge of typhoid bacilli, but they understood basic principles of bacteriology. They controlled the spread of infection simply by practicing and urging on their male coworkers, with limited success, basic hygiene. In so doing, they freed doctors to do more doctoring without taking time to address nursing activities. Unlike the filthy and resentful recruits assigned to the hospital tents, the nurses cleaned bedpans and urinals and saw that basins of vomit were not dumped at the entrance to the sick tents.[62]

Beyond the critical hygienic aspect of trained nursing, it is difficult to stipulate the professional skills of the American nurses of 1898. Unlike their Civil War predecessors, Spanish-American War nurses assigned to hospitals in Cuba could stay "busy taking temps and pulse."[63] But entirely like Civil War nurses, they drove themselves to exhaustion, illness, and occasionally death trying to keep infected and wounded soldiers alive with supportive care. Moldy hardtack and worm-infested bread were mercifully gone. But nurses struggled to provide the wounded with linen and night shirts, and for those unable to eat solids, they combed camps and harangued officials for milk, broth, and eggs. For those delirious with fever or suffering from head wounds, they searched for ice and described the correct manner of preparing and applying ice compresses.[64] This was all in the service of supportive care, if only in the effort to obviate criminal neglect, such as that reported by one Louis E. Kreuss, a private in the ninth New York regiment. Kreuss told the postwar Dodge Commission that "he went for four days in the hospital without medicine or food and that another soldier died of typhoid and was left for two days without being moved." Fannie Dennie, a graduate nurse assigned to Leiter General Hospital, to which patients from the Camp Thomas field hospitals were sent, reported that arriving patients had the worst bedsores she had ever seen and looked as if they had not had water near them for weeks.[65]

What else was there? In his retrospective *Medico-Surgical Aspects of the Spanish American War*, published in 1900, Nicholas Senn, who served in Cuba as chief surgeon of the Sixth Army Corps, devoted a chapter to "Nurses and Nursing in the War" without saying anything about what exactly the nurses did of a professional nature. To the contrary, he recurs to the Nightingalean assumption that Anita McGee and her associates worked so hard to overcome. Among the male soldiers selected for nursing duty, he mused with profound understatement, many "lacked entirely the necessary qualifications by nature and training for such an important and responsible position."[66] And what does Senn mean by "qualification by nature"? Having nothing at all to say about nurses' professional skills, he recurred to the timeworn Nightingalean platitudes, opining that nursing

> is woman's special sphere. It is her natural calling. She is a born nurse. She is endowed with all the qualification, mentally and physically, to take care of the sick. Her sweet smile and gentle touch are often of more benefit to the patient than the medicine she administers. The dainty dishes she is capable of preparing, as a rule, accomplish more in the successful treatment of disease than drugs.[67]

If there is more to military nursing in the Spanish-American War, Senn is either ignorant of it or chooses to keep it to himself. He is quick to remind readers of the medical improvements enjoyed by American soldiers—of how the septic moist compresses of the Civil War were replaced with antiseptic occlusive dressings—and he lists the various antiseptics available to surgeons: iodoform, salicylic acid, carbolic acid, mercuric chlorid [sic], zinc chlorid [sic], and salol.[68] First-aid kits intended for distribution among the troops in Cuba and the Philippines proved too bulky to carry into the field but still "did excellent service in the field hospitals." The kits comprised "two antiseptic compresses of sublimated gauze in oiled paper, one antiseptic sublimated cambric bandage, with safety-pin, one triangular Esmarch bandage with safety pin."[69]

But where did the training of the nurses enter into all this? Did they prepare the widely used "sublimate gauze," i.e., gauze impregnated with a 1:1000 solution of the potent and poisonous antiseptic mercury bichloride? Were they specifically trained in the preparation and application of different dressings, including the selection of antiseptic powders, ointments, and liquids for different kinds of wounds? Did they exercise independent judgment in other medical aspects of wound management, or did they receive explicit orders from surgeons on how to dress the wounds of this or that patient?

Individual nurses no doubt did some or all of these things—by 1898 military hospitals had established the same hierarchical nursing system as civil hospitals[70]—but absent any kind of protocol or reminiscences about nursing practice in general, many nurses probably did less rather than more. Patients in Camp Thomas who were transferred to the newly opened Sternberg Field Hospital in the summer and fall of 1898 had all been given doses of calomel (to clear the bowels) and jalop (to induce vomiting), presumably by army nurses.[71] No doubt the hospital nurses all kept morphine on hand for soldiers who required it, but then Civil War nurses likewise administered chloroform and opium without "prescription" when they felt it necessary.[72] In short, the skill set of American and American-trained nurses into the twentieth century—excepting only their understanding and application of bacteriology—appears much closer to that of Civil War nurses than to the nurses of the cataclysmic world war that lay ahead.

Things were little different, nursing-wise, for the British and British colonial nurses tending Boer War casualties a year later. For nurses and the orderlies they supervised, it was again a matter of supportive care, especially for soldiers struck down with typhoid, malaria, dysentery, and yellow fever. According to Alice Bron, a Belgian Red Cross nurse serving in South Africa with a Dutch-Belgian hospital unit, soldiers with typhoid fever, then in military camps, typically had their own hospitals, lest they infect beds intended for the wounded. Of course, such preventive measures were impossible on the ambulance trains that shuttled the wounded and infected together to hospitals.[73]

In their own tiny hospitals,[74] typhoid patients, like those in the Spanish-American War, received ice-caps, sponge baths, and cold packs to bring down their fever. But ice, as in Cuba, Puerto Rico, and the Philippines, was often in short supply, and nurses welcomed the occasional hailstorm that enabled them to collect and use hail stones to cool their patients.[75] Those typhoid patients whose condition was complicated by pneumonia also received poultices, whereas those with hemorrhages received ergotine, a powerful alkaloid extracted from a fungus that grows on cereals, to control the bleeding.[76] Many of the treatments were administered by orderlies. The supervising Sisters who belonged to the Army Medical Service played very little role in patient care. By all accounts, they simply distributed medicines and stimulants (diluted brandy and strychnine, among them) for the orderlies to administer; the more numerous civilian nurses often did so themselves, over the protests of the army sisters. Stimulants were an essential part of any hospital stay. At Ladysmith Hospital in the KwaZulu-Natal province, an anonymous "Sister X" reported patients were often given two or three stimulants at the same time, so that many "were undoubtedly on the verge of D.T., trembling like aspen leaves in consequence."[77]

Bedside wound management during the Boer War involved the collaboration of surgeons and orderlies. Simply preparing for the surgeon's morning visit was an elaborate affair, which summoned the kind of turn-of-the-century nursing skill relegated to orderlies. I. S. Inder, a trained orderly serving at No. 1 General, a 1,000-bed base hospital in Wynberg, itemized the steps of the process in his memoir of 1903. Prior to the surgeon's bedside visit he prepared swabs of absorbent wool, Boracic gauze and Boric wool along with the "strapping" and "sticking" plaster needed to affix them; then he sterilized the case of operating instruments; then he readied antiseptics such as iodoform and Boric powder; then he put waterproof sheeting under the patient; and finally he made sure the dressing tray and waste bucket were in place. With the surgeon's arrival, wound dressing "became a series of unbandaging, swabbing off old dressing, examination and pressing of punctures, syringing, powdering with antiseptics, and application of fresh dressing and bandages." Elsewhere Inder is clear that orderlies "have to bear a hand in re-dressing the wounds" and that he himself had "syringed" a patient's open wounds at bedside throughout the day.[78]

• • •

Accounts of nurses and orderlies who served in the Spanish-American and Boer Wars speak to the evolutionary growth in nursing practice in the decades that followed the Civil War. The growth was expressed in a small number of new nursing activities, like taking and recording temperature and pulse and applying more elaborate wound dressings. Still, the new nurse of the late 1890s remained ensnared in mechanical and often menial work that, despite the efforts of Anita McGee and her colleagues, remained true to the Nightingalean vision of nursing into which these nurses were trained and socialized. Understanding the importance of hygiene in preventing the spread of bacterial infection reflects a basic understanding of bacteriology, certainly, but it gained expression in mundane house-cleaning and body-cleaning chores. Similarly, learning how to irrigate open wounds and prepare different kinds of antiseptic dressings are skills, but not the kind of skills we impute to professionals. There is no specialized knowledge involved here, nothing inaccessible to people outside the nursing profession who are able to follow sequential instructions with care. Even the antiseptic dressings available to nurses and nursing orderlies—the basic tools of the bedside—had, with the exception of iodoform, been around for some time. Boric acid, carbolic acid, and salicylic acid, for example, had all been developed in the 1870s. The nurses also used mercury chloride, whose use dates back to Arab physicians of the Middle Ages.[79] The single piece of recently invented technology available just in time for these two wars was the Roentgen ray or "x-ray" apparatus, and nurses played no role in its use, which required medically trained experts.[80]

It was the First World War that finally pushed nursing into a new operational orbit. The battlefield nursing of 1914–1918, that is, changed altogether what it meant to be a trained nurse and to provide intensive nursing care. In so doing, the Great War was the historical site of what the historian Thomas Kuhn famously termed a paradigm shift.

The military nurses of America were poised for this change; their hospital training and organizational gains since the Civil War undergirded this change. And their nursing work during the Spanish-American War and, for the Brits and Canadians, the Boer War, primed them for it. But it was the Great War that was the tipping point.

How did the paradigm shift in nursing care come about? The Great War, in all its inglorious, destructive mechanization, created heretofore unimagined kinds of calamitous injury and prolonged dying. When the war broke out in 1914, military medicine was thoroughly scientific, but the science fell short of these injuries, both surgically and medically. Surgeons performed operations that were as effective as their armamentarium permitted, and all told they achieved remarkable success keeping patients alive long enough to begin an uncertain postsurgical odyssey back in the wards. There are surgical heroes aplenty in the Great War, pushing the outside of the envelope of their craft as they operated nonstop for 15, 24, even 36 hours in the rushes that followed major battles. Yet, in a paradox all too familiar to historians of medicine, their heroic operations pushed the boundaries of what was surgically possible at the expense of life-altering and life-threatening complications that someone—but not the surgeons—had to manage.

In the casualty clearing stations and field hospitals of the Western front, there were no attending physicians or residents to assess patients

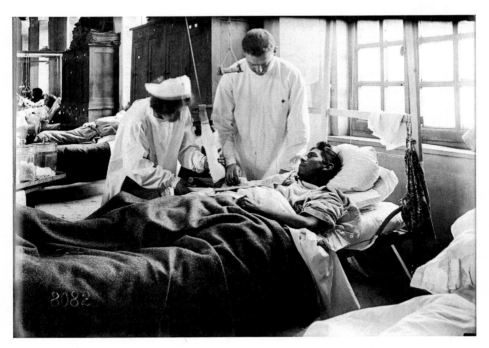

An American Red Cross nurse tends to a wounded Native American soldier from Michigan at ARC Hospital No. 41, St. Denis, 1918 (Library of Congress).

for surgery or provide postsurgical care. It was nurses who did the triaging that determined which soldiers made it to the operating table sooner, later, or not at all, just as it was nurses who provided postsurgical care, which was often prolonged, complicated, and procedural in nature. It also included, on occasion, bedside surgery.

It was no different with new battlefield-related nonsurgical injury, including all manner of localized and systemic infection. Surgeons usually provided initial assessments of the medical cases, just as, stepping outside their operative role, they assessed soldiers whose bodies were unscathed but whose minds had given way to symptoms of "shell shock" or to madness altogether. And they evaluated, diagnosed, and prescribed treatment for victims of infectious disease, from trench fever and trench foot to dysentery and measles to the deadly influenza of 1917. But for all these conditions, it was the nurses who provided most of the actual care, which could involve, inter alia, choice and schedule of medications, management of complicated wounds, devising and utilizing orthopedic devices, and providing physical therapy and supportive psychotherapy.

None of which implies that the nurses of World War I did not provide support, comfort, and reassurance as their schedules and their stamina permitted. The work of Anita McGee and her cohort notwithstanding, they were caring Nightingalean nurses by disposition. In terms of how the nurses came to think of themselves, however, this dimension of their work was subordinated to the medicalized rigors of nursing practice, especially during the rushes of incoming wounded that followed battles. In this sense, the American nurses of the Great War handed Anita McGee her final victory, since they demonstrated with finality that nursing care, however compassionate in tone and tenor, was indeed a matter of scientific expertise and not Nightingalean sentiment.

Nor do their epiphanies, whether as moments, interludes, or existential turning points, detract from this achievement. On the contrary, epiphanies of disillusionment, horror, and disgust only heighten it, since they attest to the skeptical self-awareness that is an aspect of professional maturation—and the ability to labor on, as professionals do, despite it. For health care professionals, scientific expertise is followed, necessarily, by painful awareness of the limits of this expertise in the realm of clinical praxis. And for many it brings in its wake a more insistent, even intrusive, need to justify the ends to which this expertise, whatever its limitations, is being deployed by others. This responsibility, which intensifies among battlefield nurses, is a deeply personal matter that cannot be captured in codes of professional ethics, regarding which American graduate nurses lagged far behind other professions in any event.[81] Yet, just such responsibility is, or at least ought to be, part of any health care professional's coming of age in a time of war.

The chapters to follow flesh out these broad claims both figuratively and corporeally by examining the different ways in which American nurses, working alongside other allied nurses and volunteer assistant nurses (VADs),[82] responded to clinical contingencies and inadequate medical staff with skill, imagination, resourcefulness, and boldness. Like the nurses of earlier wars, they nursed on, but they did so in realms of procedural intervention—medical, surgical, orthopedic, and psychiatric—unknown to their predecessors. That they did so, typically with the blessing of medical colleagues, reflects both the state of nursing skill and nursing professionalism in the second decade of the last century. With the skill set and strengthened professionalism came the readiness to carry out doctors' orders, certainly, but also, when circumstances required, the ability to exercise independent *medico-nursing* judgment. Without nurses capable of such judgment, especially in the face of draconian injuries far beyond the prewar experience of doctors and nurses alike, World War I might well have followed a different timeline.

This perspective on military nursing in World War I differs from traditional approaches to nursing history. Rather than looking at the nurses biographically or organizationally or refracting their wartime role through the lens of gender and the ongoing struggle for women's rights, it places the actualities of nursing practice on the Western front in the foreground. We want to look outward from different kinds of wounds, injuries, and infections to the nurses who took into their wards soldiers who were so wounded, injured, or infected. This approach enables us to revisit the nurses through a medical lens that focuses on the actual clinical work they performed. In so doing, it demonstrates how the history of medicine can enlarge our understanding of the emergence of modern nursing practice at the same time as it deepens our appreciation of what this particular cohort of nursing professionals, these gallants of the Great War, were able to accomplish.

2

Blood

"Oh the pitiful sights"[1]

Now the term bloodbath is used metaphorically, even in its wartime sense of a bloody massacre in which lives are lost. Often it is used more loosely still, as in the crushing of opponents in sports, business, or politics, or the purging of employees at a company. "There Could Be a Bloodbath in Sports Media," declares a recent headline. "Democrats are in the Middle of a Bloodbath," reads another. "Indian IT Workers Brace for Bloodbath as Industry Veers Towards Jobless Growth," announces a third.[2]

For the nurses of the Great War working in the casualty clearing stations (CCSs) and field hospitals on the Western front, however, blood bath could take on a startling literality. Here is Beatrice Hopkinson writing in the fall of 1917 at the height of the third battle of Ypres (hereinafter 3rd Ypres or Passchendaele), after a general hospital close to her own took a direct hit. She and an orderly began washing sheets and bedding of the bombed-out hospital in a big bath tub: "Soon we seemed to be dabbling in a sea of blood. When the lights were allowed on we looked at one another and we, too, looked as though we had been in a slaughterhouse. Our clothing was blood stained up to our chins; arms and faces too." Things could be worse still in the operating room, which during major rushes became "a slaughter house," a blood bath where ambulance drivers, aiding the exhausted nurses, "would seize a mop and pail and swipe up some of the blood from the sloppy floor, or even hold a leg or arm while it was sawn off."[3]

World War I is about wounds, a nondescript covering term that embraces the mutilation, dismemberment, and disfiguration that nurses referred to as "ghastly" wounds or "gaping" wounds—cavities of "mangled and shattered flesh where the wounds are filled with mud, torn clothing and shrapnel."[4] American nurses on the Western front were wound managers who treated ghastly, gaping wounds as a matter of course and, during the rushes that followed battles, a matter of daily routine.

Wound management began in the reception hut or tent. Hours before the fate of wounded soldiers was decided, it was nurses—not emergency room physicians or combat-trained EMS providers—who triaged incoming wounded, determining which soldiers required immediate surgery; which immediate stabilization for shock; which a ward bed to sleep and await treatment; and which quiet removal to the moribund tent to die. Surgeons, who during battle rushes could be operating up to 24, occasionally 36 hours, with only short breaks for meals, had little to do with the process. It fell to the trained nurses to deploy what resources they had to do the sorting, and then to stabilize as quickly as possible those wounded who could be stabilized.

What resources were at hand? The nurses had their eyes, which told them at once which soldiers would not survive without immediate surgery. Those with gaping wounds—the massive chest wounds, blown-open abdomens, lacerated deep tissue wounds, severe head wounds, smashed limbs oozing blood from severed vessels—were sent to the surgical hut post haste.[5] But a finer clinical judgment otherwise determined the fate of the wounded, and whether stabilization in the reception hut should be undertaken. They also prioritized among patients in need of surgery but whose condition was not dire. Who would later be brought to the surgeon and in what order? The nurses alone decided.

• • •

The wounded in this war, no less than in the Civil War, arrive off the battlefield in terrible shape: filthy, cold, dehydrated, bleeding. Many have been waiting on battlefields or in trenches for up to five days for help to arrive. So the nurses cut away what is left of their clothes and clean their cleanable wounds of dried blood, filth, dirt, and lice. For those whose wounds are not gaping, the bath house is given a speedy visit.[6] These ambulatory wounded are cleaned, warmed, and rehydrated.

But it is 1917 not 1863, so the triage nurses are faced with more complicated and pressing issues. Twenty-two years earlier, in 1895, the St. Louis surgeon George Crile performed ground-breaking research on surgical shock that led to publication of *Experimental Research into Surgical Shock*; its sequel, *Blood Pressure in Surgery*, followed in 1903.[7] The triage nurses are all too familiar with the life-threatening drop in blood pressure that followed massive blood loss, whether in surgery or through traumatic injury; the reception hut nurses are only concerned with the latter, which they refer to as "wound shock." Absent blood pressure meters and stethoscopes, much less the ability to begin blood transfusions, the nurses seek to stabilize patients in wound shock through a variety of ameliorative measures.

In her textbook of 1917, *Surgical Nursing in War*, Elizabeth Roxana Bundy, a Philadelphia physician and former superintendent of the Connecticut Training School for Nurses, provides frontline nurses with something approaching a protocol. The text is modern sounding; in 1917, it is as modern as resources of time and place permit. Make sure patients in shock are warm and dry, she enjoins. Elevate the foot of their beds to send blood toward the heart; administer morphine for severe pain; make sure aid-station bandages are not too tight or dressings dry and irritating. She alerts nurses to the fact that compound fractures of the thighbone or femur, when disturbed, are accompanied by shock more often than other fractures. And she cautions the nurses, be on the lookout for signs of hemorrhage, especially internal hemorrhage, which signals the patient is in extremis. Among the signs,

> the rapidly increasing pulse with diminished volume and easily compressible; the pallor of the features with cyanosis appearing, especially about the lips, eyelids, fingers; the peculiar gasping respiration caused by air hunger, the restlessness of the patient as he gasps for breath, and the fall of the body temperature. These signs all indicated the escape of a large quantity of blood be the hemorrhage external or internal.[8]

For soldiers in wound shock, reception hut nurses have another pathway to stabilization: the complicated procedure of pumping saline solution in the soldier, whether subcutaneously, intravenously, or rectally. Why complicated? After all, the resuscitative effect of intravenous saline infusion was demonstrated by the Scottish physician Thomas Latta during the cholera epidemic of 1831. Moreover, its effectiveness with conditions of shock in which severe loss of blood or fluid leaves the heart unable to pump blood throughout the body and threatens organ failure ("hypovolemic shock") was well established—if not really understood—by the 1880s.[9]

Nor did management of shock via saline infusions await World War I. It was first used, though not extensively, by British military surgeons during the Boer War.[10] But these historical particulars do not mitigate the onerous circumstances of nurses working in CCSs and field hospitals of the Western front. Soldiers to receive saline infusions must be kept warm, with the saline solution itself kept heated at around 120 degrees Fahrenheit. Air must be kept out of the infusion tubes. And the entire procedure must be performed aseptically in huts or tents that, depending on the season, were stifling or freezing. Elizabeth Bundy usefully formalizes the steps involved, stressing as well the infusion equipment that nurses must have at hand, and warning of the consequences of failing to meet the requirements for successful infusion. For intravenous infusion, for example,

> a scalpel, special needles, ligature silk and aneurysm needle, etc. are needed in addition, as well as forceps sponges, and sterile protectors, as for minor operations. The temperature of the fluid must be scrupulously maintained and the rate of the flow controlled. More than ever it is important to prevent the possibility of entrance of air into the needle, as a fatal result would probably follow.[11]

Of course, seriously wounded soldiers off the front can bleed out even before shock sets in. They badly need blood, but until the final year of the war they have little if any chance of getting it outside of the larger base hospitals. The rarity with which American nurses remark on observing or helping with blood transfusions underscores the singularity of what was then a complicated hospital-based procedure.[12]

Like most developments in history of medicine, blood transfusion has both a prehistory and a history. The prehistory begins in seventeenth-century France with the experiments of Jean-Baptiste Denys. But the modern history begins in 1906, when the fabulously inventive George Crile of Lakeside Hospital in Cleveland successfully transfused human blood from end-to-end suturing of donor to recipient veins.[13] And then a decade later, in early 1915, Crile led a volunteer unit from Lakeside Hospital to serve for three months at the

American Military Hospital (*Ambulance Américaine*), a privately funded American hospital that, with the outbreak of war, devoted itself entirely to the care of wounded French soldiers returning from the front. There, at the hospital's expanded facilities in the Paris suburb of Neuilly, the Lakeside unit gave blood transfusions according to the improved "cannula method" Crile had devised over the past decade.[14] Instead of suturing together veins, it utilized cannulae, thin tubes intended for insertion into veins, to draw blood from donor to recipient.

But in 1915 Crile and his team were volunteers from a neutral nation and had no opportunity to disseminate their new technique among French and British surgeons. When America entered the war more than two years later, blood transfusion was still rarely performed. Only when the U.S. Army Medical Corps, now joined in the struggle, sent over additional transfusion advocates, especially Boston's Oswald Robertson, did the situation begin to change.[15]

This development came late in the going, and even with Robertson's instruction, transfusion remained, according to Julia Stimson, "a complicated job under the very best of circumstances"[16] and one best limited to well-equipped base hospitals in large cities. So the reception hut nurses struggled to control external hemorrhage with what they have on hand: artery compression, tourniquets, blankets, and a variety of constrictive bandages. Skill and reaction time often determined whether soldiers even make it to the surgeons. Needless to say, the work is intensely visceral. "Hold that stump," a senior nurse ordered an assisting nurse, Drusilla Bowcott, in a CCS during 3rd Ypres, "and the poor chap must have felt dreadful because I grabbed his leg well above the knee, and as the solution of Eusol[17] and Peroxide was poured on to the stump, the pus was pouring over my hands."[18]

Following what stabilization the nurses could provide, surgical cases were rushed to the x-ray hut and then to the surgery hut attached to it. There surgeons relied on still other nurses to assist them at the operating table. These nurses (in British hospitals, the "theatre sisters") were surgical assistants and, as circumstances required, assistant surgeons; their role was the same in CCSs, field hospitals, and the base hospitals to which the wounded were sent for more extensive surgical repair. In the chaotic overflow of wounded that followed major battles, when as many as eight operating tables could be in continuous use around the clock for up to two weeks, they really had no choice. "In ten days," reported Helen Boylston from her front-line field hospital in late March 1917, "we have admitted four thousand eight hundred and fifty-three wounded, sent four thousand to Blighty [England], have done nine hundred and thirty-five operations." And then, with obvious pride, "—and only twelve patients have died."[19] "One doctor and one nurse work at each table," Julia Stimson wrote her parents from Base Hospital 21 near Rouen several months later,

> and you can imagine what surgical work the nurse has to do, no mere handing of instruments and sponges, but sewing and tying up and putting in drains while the doctor takes the next piece of shell out of another place. Then after fourteen hours of this, with freezing feet, to a meal of tea and bread and jam, and off to rest if you can in a wet bell tent in a damp bed without sheets, after a wash with a cupful of water.[20]

Even auxiliary nurses, with their very abbreviated training, were pressed into surgical duty. Kate Norman Derr, the well-off daughter of a former medical director in the U.S. Navy, was studying art in France when war broke out in 1914. Rallying to the French cause, she volunteered at local hospitals before earning a nursing certificate from the French Red Cross. In September 1915 she reported to a French field hospital in the Marne Valley where, assigned to the operating ward, she assisted surgeons in more than 25 operations performed daily. Horrified by the wounds she encountered, she nonetheless relished her newfound surgical identity. "I think you would sicken with fright if you could see the operations that a poor nurse is called upon to perform," she wrote her family. She was referring to "the putting in of drains, the washing of wounds so huge and ghastly as to make one marvel at the endurance that is man's, the digging about for bits of shrapnel. I assure you that the word responsibility takes a special meaning here." For Derr, it was the struggle itself, "the sense that one is saving bits from the wreckage," that managed to sequester the ever-present sense of being "mastered by the unutterable woe."[21]

Surgical technique was taught to nurses by surgeons, who then relegated certain aspects of complex multi-wound operations to them. Shell fragments and shrapnel often lodged in different parts of a soldier's body, in which case surgeons concentrated on the most penetrative, life threatening wounds while the nurses, forceps in hand, dealt with those that were manageable, if far from minor. Sometimes, during major rushes of wounded, there was simply no time to teach technique so it was simply coaxed out of the attending nurse. This was the case with May Tilton, an Australian nurse assigned to a surgical team at CCS No. 3 near Poperinghe during 3rd Ypres. The surgeon to nurse Tilton: "Get on with the minor wounds, sister, or we won't save this chap." When Tilton demurred, pointing out she had never before performed such work, he advised her to "forget yourself and think only of our patients."[22]

If surgeons taught nurses the rudiments of surgical technique, it was American nurses who administered the general anesthesia that made surgery possible and, having mastered the technique, taught it to other nurses and physicians.

•   •   •

The elevation of trained nurses to expert anesthetists began in the final decade of the nineteenth century, when William Mayo of Rochester, Minnesota, soon to become the eminent "Dr. Will" of the Mayo Clinic, trained his nurse and future wife, Edith Graham, to administer chloroform during his operations. Then, after their marriage in 1893, he hired Alice Magaw and later Florence Henderson to replace her. Magaw and Henderson became master anesthetists, and their expertise was not lost on surgeons visiting the Mayo Clinic. Over the next two decades other eminent surgeons followed the Mayos' practice and hired gifted nurses to serve as their personal anesthetists, making sure their hospitals provided all the supplementary training and operating room experience the nurses required. The best known among them was none other than George Crile. In 1908 he "annunciated" to Agatha Hodgins, the hospital's head nurse, the special role for which he had chosen her.[23]

These pioneer nurse anesthetists in turn trained other nurses, interns, and visiting physicians in anesthesia technique. Such training, almost always provided by apprenticeship and observation, had become necessary at the large hospitals of the day—New York's Presbyterian and Massachusetts General, among them—owing to the need to provide an anesthesia service for hospital surgeons who could not brook delay in performing their daily scheduled procedures. The training of student nurse anesthetists by senior nurse anesthetists occurred at a time when administration of anesthesia was not yet part of the medical school curriculum; nor were hospital interns on the floor, always on the go, interested in learning to become competent anesthetists.

This proved to be just as well, since surgeons quickly realized that it was nurses and not interns who by temperament and aptitude were better suited to become staff anesthetists. Nurses, they believed, would give undivided attention to the anesthetized patient, whereas interns would likely divide their attention between the patient and the surgery being performed. In the five years leading up to the Great War, the role of nurses as anesthetists of choice won broad acceptance among physicians and hospital administrators. Such acceptance, be it noted, was freighted with gendered assumptions that extolled the superior aptitude of women for nursing in general.[24]

The training provided by senior nurse anesthetists to hospital staffs, as noted, attracted visiting nurses and physicians to observe and learn. Before the outbreak of World War I, their informal training clinics evolved into the first postgraduate courses in anesthesia administration at St. Vincent's Hospital in Portland, Oregon (1909), St. John's Hospital in Springfield, Illinois (1912), New York Post-Graduate Hospital (1912), and Long Island College Hospital in Brooklyn (1914).[25]

It was Alice Magaw who, shortly after her appointment to Mayo-run Saint Mary's Hospital in 1893, perfected the method of open-drop anesthesia, then popular in Germany, in which ether or chloroform was slowly dripped, rather than poured, onto a gauze-covered mask placed over the patient's face. Her results with the method, which she began publishing in regional medical journals in 1899, attested to her utter mastery of the technique. Her results were astounding: Of 993 operations performed with the open-drop method in 1899 alone, she reported no anesthesia-related accident or need for artificial respiration.[26] By 1908, however, the open-drop method was being replaced by a superior method of inducing general anesthesia: the combination of nitrous oxide and oxygen. With this transition came the complicated apparatus for combining the two gases in a manner that maintained deep sleep—long a problem with the use of nitrous oxide alone—while preventing the lack of oxygen (anoxia) that resulted in tissue damage or worse—a second problem long associated with nitrous oxide.

It was a tall order and required technical skill far beyond that associated with oral administration of ether or chloroform. The ratio of oxygen to nitrous oxide had to be continuously adjusted via pressure regulators and a regulating valve based on visual and aural assessment of the patient's breathing patterns. From time to time, moreover, vapors from a heated cup of ether or chloroform had to be added to the mix to preserve deep sleep. In 1910, Graham Clarke, founder of the Ohio Chemical Company, designed the Ohio Monovalve, one of the most successful early anesthesia machines for administering the mix; his collaborator was none other than Agatha Hodgins.

In 1915 during George Crile's three-month stint in Neuilly, he and his Lakeside Hospital staff demonstrated the superiority of nitrous oxide-oxygen anesthesia to the staff of the American Hospital. The demonstration came at an opportune time, as the hospital staff was by then coping with war casualties who, owing to massive blood loss,

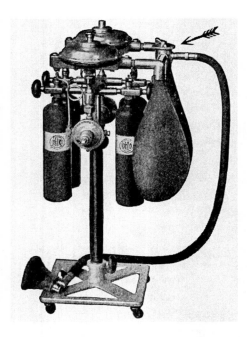

The Ohio Monovalve, one of several gas anesthesia machines used in field hospitals during World War I. William Harper De Ford, *Lectures on General Anaesthetics in Dentistry* ([Pittsburgh: Lee S. Smith, 1912], 116).

often arrived in shock. Needless to say, Agatha Hodgins was by his side, administering anesthesia for Crile's operations and instructing staff on the new technique involved.

The same was true of other nurse anesthetists who followed Miss Hodgins in the months leading up to America's entry into the war. Gertrude Garrard, who became Harvey Cushing's nurse anesthetist in 1916, accompanied him to France as part of the Harvard unit, which formed Base Hospital No. 5. On arrival, however, the unit was assigned to British General Hospital No. 11 in Camiers, just south of the Belgian village of Ypres. There Cushing, whose reputation as a head and brain surgeon preceded him, was immediately assigned to British CCS 46 in anticipation of the Passchendaele offensive soon to be launched. So Cushing was off to Ypres with a small team that comprised a nurse, an orderly, and of course Miss Gerrard. From July 22 through November 1, Cushing and Gerrard operated on 219 soldiers with head wounds, of which 133 involved the brain. "They think I'm killing Miss Gerrard," he remarked to staff members from the adjacent hospital who came to observe his operations in early August. "She does double work—anesthetist and instruments too—moreover, like me, has no regular schedule of hours."[27]

Miss Gerrard's workload did not lighten after Passchendaele. On rejoining Base Hospital No. 5, she and one other nurse anesthetist, Mary Wright, provided anesthesia for all the Harvard surgeons. When the unit relocated to Boulogne in the winter of 1918, moreover, the two nurse anesthetists found time to train nurses from Canada, New Zealand, and Australia in anesthesia technique.[28] Nor were Harvard's nurse anesthetists unique in their obligation to train others. The British, who entered the war relying on physician anesthetists, were immediately struck by the competence of the American nurses. The two nurse anesthetists at the University of Pennsylvania's Base Hospital No. 10, Florence Burkey and Anna Murphy, were especially admired, and from early spring of 1918 through spring of 1919, small classes of British and Canadian nurses received anesthesia training at Penn's base hospital. No less a British surgeon than Berkeley Moynihan sent his anesthetist to Agatha Hodgins for training.[29]

Shortly after America entered the war in April 1917, the U.S. Surgeon General's office declared nitrous oxide-oxygen the preferred method of inducing general anesthesia; the directive meant that army hospitals were equipped with the new generation of anesthesia gas machines.[30] Self-evidently, the nurse-anesthetists would be pressed into service both at home and abroad. Many of them trained military nurses stateside; others joined their hospital units overseas where they continued to provide anesthesia service for the base hospital surgeons while training others in the use of the new nitrous oxide-oxygen gas machines.

The U.S. Navy, for its part, did not wait for America's entry into the war. Beginning in December 1916 it established a three-month program in anesthesia for navy nurses at Pennsylvania Hospital, where they trained under Emma Fraser, the hospital's nurse anesthetist. The army too appreciated the need for expert nurse anesthetists but only instituted its own training program after America's

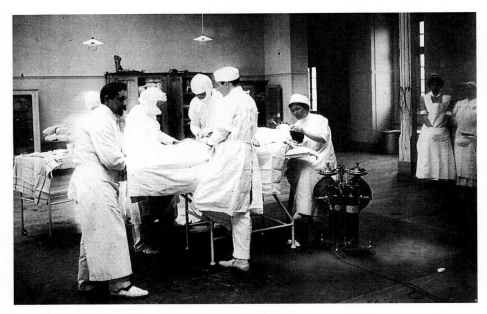

Agatha Hodgins administering anesthesia at the American Ambulance Hospital in Neuilly-sur-Seine, just outside Paris. Hodgins came to France in 1915 with George Crile's Lakeside Hospital Unit from Cleveland (reprinted with permission of the American Association of Nurse Anesthetists).

entry into the war. In April and then again in September 1918, it sent small groups of army nurses to Saint Mary's Hospital in Rochester, Minnesota, where they completed a six-week course of instruction led by Mary Hines, then William Mayo's personal anesthetist.[31]

It bears noting that all nurses, not just those destined to become nurse anesthetists, received training in anesthesia by the beginning of the twentieth century. This proved critically important. All nurses serving in CCSs and field hospitals near the front—not just those with additional training and assigned to surgical services—could be called on to provide anesthesia by the open-drop method during the rushes that followed major battles and kept surgeons operating around the clock. The notebook of Alma Adelaide Clarke speaks to this expectation.

Born in Paris in 1890 to a Parisian mother and an American father, Clarke cared for orphans throughout France through the Committee Franco-America for the Protection of the Children of the

Frontier. During the final days of the war and for the first half of 1919, however, she accepted reassignment as an Auxiliary Nurse at American Red Cross (ARC) Military Hospital No. 1 in Neuilly-sur-Seine. Her notebook of November 1918 preserves the instructions she and her cohort received in France by the ARC prior to receiving their nursing assignment. Anesthesia, Clarke recorded,

> is a poison of the nervous system: 1. Chloroform 2. Ether 3. Chlorine of ether. Local: 1.Cocaine 2. Ice 3. Chloride d'ethyl
>
> Keep chloroform and ether away from the sun. Have 10 ____ bottles on hand for operation. Ether *very* inflammable.
>
> Preparation for anesthesia: fasting in morning ... neck on bolster, Use *pince á longue* [long tweezers] to hold back tongue ... oxygen ... see case of accident
>
> Take wire cone, place linen over, then rubbing (?) outside and inside ether large spoonful on flannel [Funnel?].

And elsewhere in her notebook:

> To anesthetize: rub face with Vaseline. Put teaspoon of chloroform on handkerchief [hakf] use *pince à longue* to hold back tongue, Oxygen here cause of accident ... tell patients to breathe and not lie afraid. Watch breathing when patient.... Ether: Not dangerous as chloroform for heart but congests lungs.[32]

• • •

The critical role of World War I nurses on surgical teams, where they assumed the responsibilities of surgical assistants and assistant surgeons, is far removed from their role in the operating tents of earlier nineteenth-century wars. During the Civil War, Missourian Mary Ellis, who raised a Union regiment with her husband, was one nurse who did pick up the scalpel, especially during the Battle of Pea Bridge in March 1862. There, she recalled 30 years later, she "stood at the surgeon's table, not one or two, but many hours, with the hot blood steaming into my face." But the role she assumed was an emergency measure undertaken in the heat of battle, when unattended casualties quickly became fatalities. And even during such emergencies, when speeding up the surgeon's operative work was nurses' urgent charge, they found the work difficult, at first repugnant. Ellis, for example, recalled how "nature rebelled against such horrible sights" and she fainted, only to return to the operating table when she was able to.[33]

Clara Barton similarly assisted in surgery at the battles of Antietam and Fredericksburg in the fall of 1862. At Antietam, moreover, in a farmhouse just off the main battlefield, she famously performed a minor operation on her own. Confronted with a very young soldier with a bullet lodged in his cheek, she took out her pocketknife and, with the assistance of a wounded orderly who held the boy's face immobile, she cut out the bullet, then washed and dressed the wound. To be sure, the boy had begged Barton to do the operation, knowing the wait for a surgeon's attention would be intolerably long.[34] But the fact is that Barton's surgery was a success. And then three months after Fredericksburg, in March 1863, the Union nurse Emily Parsons, working at Benton Barracks Hospital outside St. Louis, asked a kindly surgeon to operate on the harelip of a black child brought to the hospital. The surgeon assented, which led Parsons to muse, "I suppose I shall assist."[35] In what way, one wonders, would she have assisted?

No doubt other examples of nurse surgery during the Civil War can be found, but they remain rare exceptions to the rule. Most often, Civil War nurses "assisted" surgeons by providing postoperative care with varying degrees of independence. Simply releasing a patient after surgery to a nurse's care was a mark of trust on the surgeon's part that rarely escaped notice. "Yesterday," wrote Parsons from an earlier posting at the Union hospital at Fort Schuyler, New York, "I had two cases sent to me from the operating room.... The Doctor trusted Me enough to send me Number One without coming himself, though it was the first time I have had an operation of any extent here."[36]

The small body of nurse reminiscences from the brief Spanish-American War of 1898 and the lengthy Anglo-Boer War of 1899–1902, respectively, suggests that, if anything, nurses were less active in the surgical realm than during the Civil War. The reason, in part, is that both were less wars of battlefield injury than of systemic infection—yellow fever, dysentery, malaria, typhus, measles, gastroenteritis, and especially typhoid, which felled soldiers, nurses, and lay populations alike in both wars.[37] In the 31-month Anglo-Boer War, 22,000 British soldiers were treated for wounds, but 20 times that number were hospitalized for disease. The British lost roughly 14,000 soldiers to disease compared to 5,000 killed in action. The numbers are far lower in the three-and-a-half-month Spanish-American War of 1898, but the ratio much the same. Typhoid alone killed 1,580 men while only 243 died in action.[38]

Nurse reminiscences from both wars are mainly stories of infectious illness and the ward conditions under which it was treated. Wound management is occasionally recounted, but less to explain nurse activities than to relate the stressful environment in which nurses labored. Conflicts were especially rife in the Boer War— between military and civilian nurses, military nurses of different nationalities, graduate nurses and nursing aides, and especially among military nurses, civilian nurses, and orderlies. And the conflicts and tensions of ward management travelled right up the ranks. Alice Brun, the Belgian Red Cross nurse who cared for British and Boer soldiers alike during the Boer War, provided wound care under the supervision of surgeons of different nationalities. No sooner had she completed a series of complicated hip-thigh dressings, as instructed by an English surgeon, than she was ordered by his German counterpart to cut away all her "elaborate bandages" and redo them in *his* prescribed manner. She did so under the reproachful stares of the poor patients.[39]

On the Western front of the Great War, on the other hand, the complex wound management that followed surgery was usually in nurses' hands, and there is little evidence of conflicts among surgeons under the same roof (or tent) as to how they should go about it. Their work began back in the reception hut, where nurses determined which wounds required a surgeon's postoperative attention and which they could handle themselves. For smaller wounds—the term being relative—nursing care segued into surgical care. Nurses irrigated wound beds with saline solution and then debrided them, using sterile probes to locate and remove shrapnel, bone fragments, embedded clothing, and debris. Finally, they dressed wounds with the antiseptics of the day—iodine, carbolic acid, hydrogen peroxide, perchloride of mercury, sodium hypochlorite, boracic acid, salicylic acid, chloride of zinc, potassium permaganate. Antiseptics could be given either alone or in combination, in liquid or paste form. Given the plethora of options and known toxicity of the more effective antiseptics, choosing the optimal dressing for a particular soldier was no simple matter. For soldiers with large and deep infected open wounds—the "gaping wounds" or "horribly bad wounds" or "wounds so huge and ghastly" of which the nurses wrote[40]—there was a novel and promising approach to antiseptic therapy, and nurses were at the heart of it.

• • •

Nurses and surgeons of the Great War are children of the era of Listerian antisepsis. They know all about bacteria and the speed with which deep open wounds turn septic. In all previous wars, badly infected wounds usually meant automatic amputation, frequent rein-fection, and frequent death. But now, two scientists, Alexis Carrel and Henry Dakin, have stretched the first-generation Listerian approach to its curative limit and devised a new method for "steril-izing," as they say, badly infected deep wounds and saving limbs and lives.

Carrel is a French surgeon and biologist of international repu-tation. Already in 1912 he has received the Nobel Prize in Physiology or Medicine for developing a new technique for suturing blood ves-sels; he is a pioneer of vascular surgery. Dakin is a British-born chemist working at the Rockefeller Institute in New York. After the war, his research on organic compounds, including the relationship between hydrogen peroxide and amino acids, will profoundly influ-ence biochemical theory. The two meet in late 1914 in the laboratory of a field hospital near the forest of Compiègne in northern France. Both there and at temporary hospital No. 21 run by France's *Service de santé des armées* (Defense Health Service), they collaborate on a problem that is easy to conceptualize but in 1914 extremely difficult to solve. As Carrel puts it, they want to figure out a way to suppress wound infection by chemical means. They want, that is, to find a way to sterilize infected wounds through the chemicals, by which they mean the antiseptics, available to them.

They know that the antiseptic treatment of battle-inflicted infected wounds has already been considered and rejected by some of the most prominent surgeons of the time, Britain's Berkeley Moyni-han and Almroth Wright among them. Because the microbes that cause war wounds travel deep into human tissue by projectiles that carry clothing fragments, mud, and field manure with them, the sur-geons reason, they are beyond the reach of antiseptics.[41]

But Carrel and Dakin are not dissuaded. The surgeons, they believe, do not understand the exactitude with which Lister's method must be employed if it is to be successful. Indeed, the surgeons have little understanding of Listerian principles per se. Carrel and Dakin believe that antiseptic treatment *can* be effective in sterilizing (i.e., disinfecting) deep septic wounds, if only they can find the right chem-ical and devise the right delivery system. They begin with the secure knowledge that any infected wound, however deep or extensive, still begins as a local wound, so that the problem of "wound sterilization" will always be, for a time, a matter of local treatment. This fact bolsters their belief that it will yield to timely antiseptic treatment.

Dakin tackles the problem of wound sterilization. His chemical challenge is to find an antiseptic, however modified, that will be potent enough (i.e., of "sufficient bactericidal power"[42]) to kill the microorganisms causing infection without damaging and potentially destroying the surrounding healthy tissue. But the very challenge points to the possibility of a solution, since infected and healthy tissue have different chemical properties and react differently to specific chemicals. This is how Carrel frames the problem in expounding the method in 1917:

> Destruction by chemical means of the micro-organisms infecting a wound is rendered possible by the different resistances presented by the tissues equipped with a circulation, and the microbes which are found on their surface. The idea must be grasped that a given antiseptic substance, applied at a certain concentration, and during a certain time, is able to destroy microbes without damaging the normal tissues to any appreciable extent.[43]

In December 1914, after Dakin and his coworker, the pharmacist Maurice Daufresne, have experimented with over 200 chemicals, they finally have an answer: sodium hypochlorite ("hypochlorite of soda"), a salt of hypochlorous acid. To this chemical, Dakin and Daufresne add small quantities of two acids to neutralize its irritant properties without weakening its antiseptic action.[44] The result is "Dakin's solution," a chemical powerful and penetrating enough to disinfect deep wounds with only "feeble irritating qualities" for surrounding tissue and "almost nil" toxicity for the rest of the body.[45] The chemical terminology masks the utter simplicity of the solution: It is highly diluted bleach with a few additives to minimize its irritation of living tissue. A short time later, Daufresne refines the formula slightly, with the resulting Daufresne-Dakin solution achieving even better results.[46]

But there is a catch, and it resides in the exacting method of administration. The initial challenge falls to the surgeon: He must thoroughly debride (clean out) the wound, removing all dead and damaged tissue, bone fragments, shell fragments, and detritus. In the process he must sculpt the wound, to the extent possible, into a broad crater of tissue. The very small "instillation tubes" that will reach down into the wound—anywhere from two to ten or more—are carefully embedded at different locations in the wound and attached to the bedside apparatus according to Carrel's precise directions.

Carrel knows average surgeons will find the method difficult to implement, which is indeed the case. After finishing his work at his Rockefeller-funded hospital in Compiègne, he returns to America where, in the spring of 1917, he begins providing instruction on both the method and its conceptual rationale at a 100-bed War Demonstration Hospital constructed on the grounds of the Rockefeller Institute in Manhattan. So American surgeons and nurses, both military and civilian, are given a running head start in the use of the Carrel-Dakin method. At the Demonstration Hospital in New York, they acquire hands-on experience with the new method, whereas their patients are among the first beneficiaries of it. American surgeons who train under Carrel continue to find the method difficult, but they at least leave the training course with a greatly improved understanding of scientific antisepsis and the value of procedural precision. Carrel believes they will be better surgeons on account of it.[47]

As to Dakin's solution, it only sterilizes infected wounds without damaging surrounding tissue if used in a particular concentration and, further, if it remains in contact with the microbes for a "known period of time," which turns out to be, in most cases, three to five days.[48] To this end, Carrell devises a system of glass containers, clamps, and tubing that adds up to a Rube Goldberg–type siphoning device, with the whole affair held in place with bandages and an adjustable clamp on the main tube to regulate the amount of antiseptic fed into the wound at 2–3 hour intervals.

Beginning in 1915, many explanations of the Carrel-Dakin method were published in the medical literature, and demonstrations were given throughout Europe. This brief description was intended for American home front physicians who had never observed the method in operation. It is from an issue of the *Journal of the American Medical Association* a year after America's entry into the war:

> This apparatus is blown entirely of glass and fused into one compact piece. It is clean, handy and dependable. It can be made in different sizes, depending on the quantity of flushing required. The periodicity of flushing is regulated by a Hoffman pinch-cock on the tubing between the solution tank and the apparatus.

The apparatus works as follows: Solution from an irrigating bottle or bag is allowed to pass a pinch-cock [a type of valve] at a fixed rate. It accumulates in the upper chamber until it reaches the highest point of the siphon, when it suddenly is emptied by the siphon into the lower chamber. Here, by virtue of its height and its weight, it forces its way through the holes in the Carrel tube and flushes the wound. The flushing is periodic and eliminates the inconstant human element which is so often the cause of failure in the Dakin-Carrel technic.[49]

Mastering the apparatus-in-use is no easy matter, and the task falls squarely on the shoulders of the ward nurses. A matron may send newly arrived nurses to base hospitals to attend courses on the proper application of the method.[50] Back in the wards, the surgeon, assisted by a nurse, performs the initial set up. Once up and running, however, the ward nurses do all the monitoring and adjusting. They must visit the bedside of every patient receiving the treatment every several hours to release the prescribed quantity of solution from the

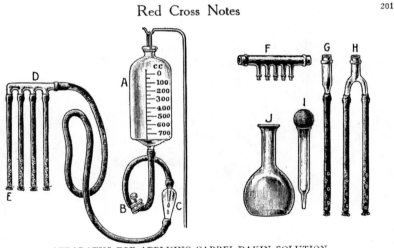

Red Cross Notes 201

APPARATUS FOR APPLYING CARREL-DAKIN SOLUTION

This apparatus is furnished by instrument dealers. Supplied by Johnson & Johnson on request.

A—Reservoir graduated.
B—Clamp for regulating flow.
C—Sight feed cup.
D—Four-way glass distributor.
E—Perforated distributing tubes with ends tied. When used for surface ends are covered with Turkish toweling.

F—Five-way glass distributor.
G—One tube glass distributor.
H—Two-way glass distributor.
I—Syringe for applying solution by hand.
J—Flask for use with syringe.

Illustration of the component parts of the Carrel-Dakin system (courtesy Johnson & Johnson Archives).

glass container affixed to the bed. They must replenish the solution at regular intervals. They must periodically inspect the surgical implant- ing of tubes to ensure uniform distribution of the solution throughout the wound. They must make sure no gauze comes between the end of each tube and human tissue. Finally, they must remove all the tubes from the wound for cleaning and resterilization every few days.[51] Until 1917, when the New Jersey manufacturer Johnson & Johnson begins producing ampoules and vials of the components of Dakin's Solution in the correct ratios, nurses prepare the solution manually, keeping to Dakin's prescribed concentration and taking pains to prepare it "in such a way that it is, and remains, substantially neutral."[52]

As late as 1918 the precision required by the method was still off- putting to surgeons, some of whom continued to advocate reliance on lesser antiseptics, such as flavine, a coal-tar derivative, that could at least be applied to wounds simply, in saturated gauze.[53] By then, though, even critics of the method ceded that, properly applied, it worked wonders, and did so because trained nurses proved capable of the great precision and attention to detail that it required. On occasion, they said as much in their journals.[54]

The image of Carrel-Dakin tubes circling down into the recesses of deep tissue concavities caused by shrapnel and shell fragments does not make for easy viewing. Nor should it. What we see in

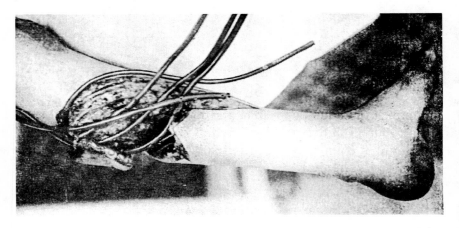

Placement of rubber Dakin tubing in a deep wound of the lower leg (G. Debaisieux, Considérations générales sur le traitement des plaies de guerre, dans l'Ambulance de "L'Océan," La Panne, s. dir. DEPAGE, A., t.1, fasc. 1, Paris, 1917).

the lower leg injury above is the unsettling reality of a wound caused by modern artillery coming up against a nascently modern technology able to prevent the amputation that would have occurred as a matter of course before the method was devised. This is the modernity, both horrid and hopeful, of the dubiously great war of 1914–1918.

In 1917, when America entered the war, blood transfusion was seldom performed, and nurses give little evidence of taking the lead in what was a base hospital procedure. Bedside Dakin-Carrel treatment, on the other hand, had become common, and here it was the newly arrived American nurses who learned from their British, Canadian, and French colleagues. A number had joined the more than 800 surgeons who had taken Carrel's courses at the Rockefeller Institute's Demonstration Hospital, but the vast majority had never encountered the method before, much less in wards full of Carrel-Dakin patients, all monitored by a single nurse. The nurses, more patient-centered than the surgeons, were quick to appreciate the seeming miracles wrought by the exotic tubular tangle as they witnessed time and again how the method saved limbs and lives. In their letters and diaries, they took time to explain the technology, however briefly, as if to justify the time and energy they expended keeping the apparatus operational.

Kate Norman Derr, writing home from her French Army Hospital near the trenches of the Marne in 1915, related with pride that her hospital's head surgeon had asked her to take charge of a ward of seriously wounded soldiers who were previously cared for by no less than Dr. Théodore Tuffier, the pioneer of cardiovascular surgery who, prior to the war, had worked at an operating table alongside Alexis Carrel. Tuffier, she recalled, "used Dakin solution to keep wound in constant bath of antiseptic and avoid amputation."[55]

After America's entry into the war, Alice O'Brien, a Minnesota lumber heiress, ambulance driver, and Red Cross floor nurse in France, wrote that most of the wounded she attended "get the Dakin treatment, a system of drains and wet bandages." Another Red Cross volunteer who came from wealth, Bostonian Isabel Anderson, was more effusive about the results of all the drains and bandages. Visiting the American Hospital in Neuilly, she wrote of Carrel-Dakin treatment: "It was wonderful to see how this simple antiseptic solution, which is at bottom nothing more than common chloride of lime [i.e., bleaching powder], healed gangrenous sores, raw wounds upon which the new cuticle would not form, or deep-seated inflammation of the bone." And later on, from Ocean Ambulance at La Panne: "The Carrel treatment with the Dakin solution is used at all the hospitals over here. There are other solutions used in certain cases, such as flavine and brilliant green, but the Carrel treatment is employed much more commonly and with great success." Elizabeth Weaver echoed Anderson about the frequency of the treatment, adding that it was in the postoperative care of soldiers with "horrible deep wounds" that Dakin's Solution played "a very important part."[56]

If nurses duly noted the wonderful benefits of the treatment, they might still complain lightly of how time-consuming it was to maintain the complicated apparatus, which included replenishing the solution and resterilizing the tubing. Ella Mae Bongard, for example, wrote of spending an entire afternoon "cleaning dirty Dakin tubes and such millions as we are using these days. All the new patients have them. It keeps one nurse busy trotting around squirting Dakin's in the tubes every hour." She hated "tramping around from house to house to make rounds and give Dakin's."[57] Isabel Anderson wrote of the hours spent preparing those Carrel tubes, "cutting the rubber tubing and puncturing them with small holes—some with a few, some with many—and tying them at the end with a string."[58]

Nor was use of the Carrel-Dakin method limited to the Western front. After the Armistice was signed, Red Cross nurses labored on throughout the world, relying on Carrel-Dakin treatment as they had during the war. One such nurse provided the *American Journal of Nursing* with a description of her postwar service at a hospital in Jerusalem. Given charge of the hospital by the occupying British, the ARC nurses treated cases of malaria and continued the local practice of treating most wounds according to Carrel-Dakin: "The native nurses say they would not know how to dress wounds without Dakin's Solution and Cerelene." And then, as if to leave no doubt whatsoever about the modernity of the native practice, she added: "Many an infected arm and leg has been saved by the Carrel-Dakin technique, and in fact I have only known of one amputation."[59]

Of course there is more to procedural intervention than Carrel-Dakin. In cases of compound fracture, nurses usually followed cleaning, irrigation, debridement, and wound dressing with splinting. Back on the wards, with a surgeon's assistance, they might begin Carrel-

Dakin treatment and monitor fractures, ever alert to obstructed circulation. Taking these nursing activities in their totality, Christine Hallett has every reason to conclude that World War I nurses emerged from their European tours as wound care practitioners, adding for good measure that in the rushes that followed major battles professional boundaries dissolved and nursing work merged with that of surgeons.[60]

Nurses of the Civil War were no less heroic, if in different ways. They were heroic simply in overcoming the resistance of surgeons and military officers to their presence right off the battlefield, where they were exposed to the naked bodies of wounded, bleeding, mutilated men. They were heroic in battling corrupt quartermasters and stewards who withheld supplies and food parcels from the wounded, not to mention racist orderlies who brutalized the wounded, especially African-Americans. And they were heroic in providing comfort care in the tradition of Florence Nightingale, struggling against the military system to keep the wounded dry, warm, and adequately fed, "mothering" them with the same compassion their granddaughters would bring to the Western front.

But Civil War nursing lacked the procedural underpinnings of Great War nursing. There was no scientific nursing to do because scientific nursing only emerged after the war. Very occasionally Civil War nurses—Clara Barton, Mary Ellis, and Emily Parsons are striking examples—would rise above the morale-sapping gender prejudice of the field hospitals and find themselves working alongside an operating surgeon. Parsons wrote of herself as a surgical nurse; with pride she related to her mother her ability to tie up a compound fracture and, as noted, anticipated being asked to assist the surgeon in repairing the harelip of a child she brought to the hospital.[61] But Parsons and others like her were by all accounts heroic exceptions to the rule. For the vast majority of Civil War nurses, authority came not from any type of training, much less from the procedural expertise it cultivated; rather, it was moral in nature and derived from the moral superiority ceded to women.

Civil War nurses also became crack administrators. In those cases in which nurses became powerful head matrons and even founders of their own field hospitals, their authority was typically wrested from surgeons and army officers who never stopped hoping the ladies would simply pack up and go home. Nurses from elite families—Hannah Ropes, Sophronia Bucklin, Kate Cumming, Clara Barton—sounded off and got results. But the results represented moral, not professional, victories. There was no system of triaging for nurses to implement; no protocol in place for cleaning and irrigating infected wounds with saline solution before applying dressings of this or that type. Nor did most surgeons encourage nurses to do anything more in the wards than prepare and serve food, provide religious solace, and write letters to loved ones for the soldiers.

•   •   •

The heroism of the nurses of World War I has to do with the manner in which they rose to their historical moment and pushed their nascent professionalism well beyond the limits set for them by their post–Civil War training programs. In so doing, they pulled into the nursing domain major developments in scientific medicine of the last quarter century. Consider the birth of bacteriology; the derivative understanding of antisepsis, asepsis, and sterilization; the development of antiseptics and serum therapy; and major advances in wound management and surgical technique. These developments, conjoined in a combat workplace that relied on collaborative staff relationships, enlarged nurses' responsibilities in a procedural direction. Unlike Civil War nurses, the nurses of the Great War initiated medical treatments, performed recently devised medical procedures, and employed recently developed medical equipment.

Nor did this expansion of the nursing role come at the expense of physicians. For one thing, the nurses enlarged their domain by mastering very recent technologies that had never become the exclusive preserve of the doctors. This pertains both to the deployment of general anesthesia, including the use of the new nitrous-oxide/oxygen units, and the Carrel-Dakin method, whose success relied on the vigilant monitoring and readjusting that only ward nurses could provide. It pertains as well to the host of diagnostic and procedural interventions triage nurses were obliged to make in the reception huts. Surgeons could not do their jobs unless nurses did theirs—this in the sense of determining as quickly as possible, with the limited resources at hand, which wounded needed immediate surgical attention, which could wait some interval of time, which required immediate stabilization after blood loss and shock, and which could be assigned to wards where they would be managed for the time being by the ward nurses. Those rushed to the x-ray and adjoining surgical tents would then be placed in the hands of nurse anesthetists, and finally handed over to surgeons who were assisted in the operating theater by surgical nurses. The demands placed on the nurses were no less than those placed on the surgeons. After the battles of Verdun and Argonne, recalled Nancy Klase, an army nurse at Base Hospital No. 42 near Neufchateau in northeastern France, the "girls" in the operating room worked a single shift that lasted two nights and three days "with no rest except to eat."[62]

These realities of life in CCSs and field hospitals during rushes of incoming casualties point to a second related reason for the enlargement of the nurse's operational domain. Surgeons had no choice but to relegate to nurses treatment, medical and surgical, of wounds that were not life threatening in the hours following evacuation from the battlefield. This reliance occurred in surgical huts as well as on wards. As operators, the surgeons relied on nurses—indeed ordered nurses—to do the "digging about for bits of shrapnel" (Kate Norman Derr) along with the surgical repair of lesser wounds so that they could concentrate on life-threatening ones.

Young American nurses such as Kate Norman Derr, from her French field hospital off the Marne, struggled to convey in letters home the enormity of what was expected of them. Their responsibilities were undertaken, it bears repeating, in the face of multiple wounds that no nurse and few if any surgeons had seen or even imagined to be see-able before the war. At times, it strained credulity even to see them as "wounds" in any remediable prewar sense. "These are not wounds, they are mush," Scottish-born Sarah McNaughtan heard a surgeon remark.[63] Edith Appleton, working out of General Hospital No. 1 Étretat, near Le Havre, wrote "of flesh torn from the thigh so deep that one could see the femoral artery or a leg so mangled that you can look quite through it in two places." Shirley Millard wrote of "faces half shot away. Eyes seared by gas; one here with no eyes at all. I can see down into the back of his head."[64] For recently minted nurses of the early twentieth century, such wounds were not merely ghastly but otherworldly, ghoulish, physically nauseating, psychologically unassimilable.

But circumstances made no allowance for inexperience or conventional sensibilities. There was no time to become hardened to bodies massacred with demonic impiety, and on those very rare occasions when a nurse confronted with horrific injuries was moved to tears, she made sure to shed them in the service tent, away from the wards and the wounded.[65] American-born Lucille Ross Jones, who eventually became a legendary Calgary nurse, began wartime nursing with only the brief training program of Britain's St. John's Ambulance Association under her belt. Initially serving in the French Red Cross in the surgical ward of *Hopital Auxiliare* No. F. 120, she recalled her first day on the job. After being taken to observe the dressing of massive wounds, she immediately began bandaging just such wounds on her own. Very soon, she was placed in full charge of dressing septic wounds. In French field hospitals in the dark days of 1915, responsibility for treating ghastly infected wounds was acquired in a matter of days.[66]

Jones's situation is hardly atypical. Indeed, the desperate condition of soldiers arriving at CCSs and field hospitals during rushes only intensified the need for newly arrived nurses to step up and become useful without delay.

> Someone thrust a huge hypodermic needle and a packet of something into my hands and told me hurriedly that every man who came in must have a shot against tetanus.... How on earth did one give a hypodermic? I'd never even *had* one. And what did "get them ready" mean?[67]

This is Shirley Millard reporting from a French field hospital in March 1918. In her case as in countless others, helpfulness quickly segued into collaboration. The entire system only worked through symbiotic collegiality among physicians, nurses, and orderlies that, with a handful of exceptions, was unimaginable during the Civil War and for which little opportunity was provided during the Spanish-American War and Boer War.

What is amazing is not only that the nurses did what was needed—the triaging, the anesthetizing, the surgical assisting, the postoperative bedside surgeries, the Carrel-Dakin applications, the complicated dressings and bandaging—but that, in the vast majority of cases, they managed to do so without forsaking the nineteenth-century Nightingalean obligation to provide care that was calming, comforting, and reassuring, especially when death was imminent. They waded through bloodbaths without flinching and patiently held the hands of dying soldiers whose faces or limbs or guts had been blown off by shell fragments. Their ability to calm and care for psychologically devastated patients, we shall see in chapter 5, often deepened into supportive psychotherapy and end-of-life counseling of a strikingly modern complexion. Arguably, psychiatric nursing was born in the CCSs and field hospitals of the Western front. In all these ways, the American nurses of World War I were clinical providers, and the well-trained nurse practitioners of our own time, licensed in many states to practice medicine (or is it "medicalized" nursing?[68]) with little or no supervision, have nothing on their gallant forebears of a century ago.

3

Total Care

"Saving bits from the wreckage"[1]

Total care began in the reception huts and included the dying as well as the living. Often the nurses sent soldiers on to the surgeons whose condition, the surgeons quickly determined, was hopeless. So they simply sent them back to the nurses, to provide what meager palliative care they could while the soldiers awaited death in the tent set aside for them, the Moribund Ward. But the nurses sometimes refused to let matters rest, recognizing that the surgeons, often operating at breakneck speed in a state of exhaustion, did not have the last word on life and death. So soldiers out of surgeons' hands might still find themselves in nurses' hands, where they were beneficiaries of nursing so intensive and prolonged that, against all odds, it segued into a curative regimen.

Kate Norman Derr, the French-trained American nurse working in a French Army Hospital near the Marne in 1915, recalled an Arab soldier who arrived at the hospital barely conscious. His seven suppurating wounds led to two successive operations, after which surgeons pronounced him hopeless and handed him back to Nurse Derr:

> It is one of the few dressings I have had that really frightened me; for it was so long, and every day for a week or more, I extracted bits of cloth and fragments of metal, sometimes at a terrifying depth. Besides my patient was savage and sullen, all that is ominous in the Arab nature. Gradually, however, the suppuration ceased, the fever fell, and suddenly one day Croya smiled.[2]

MGH-trained Helen Dore Boylston, working in the post-surgical bone ward of her Base Hospital in the winter of 1918, was no stranger to heroic surgical aftercare. Boylston enjoyed her 40 patients, and singled out a pluck Australian of over 60 with a leg "torn to pieces." "He's a Crotchety old darling, always raging and roaring about something," she wrote her family:

> One day, when I was here before, he complained of a pain in his thigh and began to run quite a temp. As his leg was laid wide open anyhow, I took a look along the bone, Dad meantime cursing the roof off. I found a walled-in pus pocket, and picking up a scalpel told Dad he'd better look out of the window for a minute, as I was going to have to hurt him. Then, before he knew what I was about, I had slit the thing open. At least two cupfuls of pus poured out, and his relief was tremendous at once. Of course his temp dropped, too. I put in a packing and watched it for a few days. It cleared up promptly. That was absolutely all.[3]

Nor did interventionist nursing end with minor bedside surgery. Nurses sometimes believed rehabilitation was possible when doctors did not, and they proved their point with paralyzed soldiers who, so the surgeons declared, would never walk again. Agnes Warner, the Canadian nurse working at the American Hospital in Neuilly, France, provides a case in point. Casualties from Alsace poured into the hospital in the spring of 1915, at which time a surgeon remarked that one of Warner's patients, her "poor paralyzed man," would never walk again. Unfazed by the pronouncement and unwilling to rest content giving the patient English lessons to help pass the time, she devised a program of rehabilitation that incorporated electrical stimulation, which only became available at the Hospital in late June. Three weeks later, she had her paralyzed man out on the balcony, where he enjoyed fresh air for the first time in six months. She was assigned another patient paralyzed from the waist down a month later, and then in mid–July she proudly reported on both patients:

> My paralyzed man stood up alone last Sunday for the first time and now he walks, pushing a chair before him like a baby. He is the happiest thing you can imagine; for seven months he has had no hope of ever walking again.... My prize patient, Daillet walks down stairs by himself now.... We are all proud of him. The doctor who sent him here from Besancon came in the other day to see how he was getting on and he could not believe it when he saw him.[4]

• • •

Among the greatest challenges for the nurses were soldiers whose gaping wounds and limbless stumps were saturated with Clostridium perfringens—soil-dwelling bacteria from the genus Clostridium that thrive in the absence of oxygen—from the heavily fertilized fields of Flanders and Northern France. These bacteria, which entered bodily cavities with the dirt, clothing, and debris picked up by bullets and exploding shell fragments, were the source of the dread gas gangrene, a condition first described by Fabricius Hildanus in a monograph of 1593, but whose identification as a distinct disease entity is generally credited to Jacque-Gilles Maisonneuve in 1853.[5]

Civil War surgeons were all too familiar with gas gangrene and struggled to locate it among then current theories of disease. Perhaps it was brought on by a constitutional weakness that resulted from exposure to bad weather, poor diet, or a poisonous "miasmatic atmosphere." Or perhaps it resulted from direct contact with the infectious matter found on sponges, washbowls, and surgical instruments.[6] Along with erysipelas, which attacked the skin and underlying tissue, it was the most feared of wound infections. Unlike infections of the more usual type that discharged thick yellow pus—the "laudable pus" that, so they believed, would drain the wound of poison and promoted healing—gangrenous infections were dry and crusty and more onerous in nature. When gangrene's characteristic symptoms accompanied large wounds in a limb, it usually meant immediate amputation at the ungloved hands of surgeons working in bacteria-infested tent hospitals. On occasion, if the amputation were performed at an early stage, before the Clostridium bacteria had spread to surrounding tissue and entered the bloodstream, the patient might survive. But by all accounts this was a serendipitous outcome. Typically, amputation of gangrenous limbs was followed by rapid reinfection and often death.

Civil War surgeons, of course, operated, literally and figuratively, without the benefit of germ theory, so their understanding could only take them so far. A promising start was made by Daniel Morgan, a Union assistant surgeon, whose study of gangrene and erysipelas was delivered to Surgeon General William Hammond in October 1862. Drawing on his experience with gangrene patients in Frederick, Maryland and West Philadelphia, he documented the dramatically reduced contagion that results when gangrene patients were removed from general wards and placed in wards of their own. There, Morgan ordered treatment with nitric acid by nurses who carefully washed their hands in a dilute chlorinated solution after dressing and bandaging wounds. The results, as he reported them, were promising.[7]

More influential still was the work of Middleton Goldsmith, a Union army surgeon stationed at Jeffersonville, Kentucky, whose *Report on Hospital Gangrene* of 1863 was issued to Union surgeons by the surgeon general. Goldsmith adopted the centuries-old Galenic assumption that wound infections of all kinds resulted from poisonous vapors in the atmosphere (miasmas) coming into contact with open wounds. As treatment, he recommended bromine and water, in both topical and injectable form. Bromine, he reasoned, was a member of the halogen family of chemicals, and other halogens, such as iodine and chlorine, had antiseptic[8] properties helpful in wound treatment. Indeed, he cited one researcher who had used iodine to neutralize the animal poison contained in rattlesnake bites. Perhaps, he reasoned, bromine would do the same with the poisonous vapors that caused gangrene. To his credit, Goldsmith urged surgeons first to cut away dead tissue and what he termed "flocculant pulp" (i.e., to debride the wound), but, given the hardness of underlying tissue and muscle, topical application of bromine, he realized, would be useless. So he recommended injecting bromine right through gangrenous "slough" or, more grisly still, pushing it through the slough with a pointed stick dipped in bromine. Pity the soldiers subjected to Goldsmith's ordeal, and lucky (perhaps) those who, prior to such treatment, pleaded intolerable pain. They at least were to receive ether or chloroform, presumably to die in peace.[9]

By the end of the nineteenth century, with Lister's germ theory firmly in place, the bacterial source of gangrenous infections finally came to light. In 1897, the Belgian biologist Emile van Ermengem isolated the type of endospore-forming microorganism that multiplied only in oxygen-free (anaerobic) conditions but it would be another quarter century until Ida A. Bengtson proposed classifying all such rod-shaped anaerobic bacteria into the genus Clostridium.

This left the nurses and surgeons of the First World War in a kind of frustrating limbo. What knowledge they had was sound, but it was also very incomplete and militated against effective treatment. They knew gas gangrene resulted from bacteria but lacked understanding of the microorganism's precise nature and mode of action. More importantly, lacking antibiotics, they were consigned to the same type of local treatments as their Civil War predecessors, abetted by an appreciation of asepsis, the availability of new and more potent antiseptics, and an ability to administer them through irrigation techniques (such as Carrel-Dakin) unavailable a half century earlier. But the progress was often inadequate to the treatment challenge before them.

Clostridium bacteria, after all, attack tissue with terrific rapidity and intensity to the point of death. We term such type of destructiveness *fulminant*, which conveys the urgency of tissue damage that is life-threatening. And Clostridium bacteria are perfidious as well, since the telltale signs of their presence may only appear days after they have attacked the body. Furthermore, these soil-dwelling bacteria not only cause the death of wound tissue; they also release toxins that cause putrefactive decay of connective tissue. It is the latter process that generates gas. Among soldiers who survived such massive bacterial assault beyond a few days, the complications were legion and sinister. They included "necrotizing fasciitis" (rapidly spreading infectious inflammation of the deep tissue [fascia] around muscles and organs), blood poisoning (pyemia, now septicemia), shock, and organ failure. Blood poisoning, a frequent complication of both gas gangrene and erysipelas, used the bloodstream to carry bacteria throughout the body; it resulted in abscesses of the brain and heart, quickly followed by death. Efforts to create a gas gangrene serum, modeled on those in use for typhoid and diphtheria, began as early as 1916, and a number of polyvalent serums (i.e., mixtures of sera from several of the microorganisms in gas gangrene) were developed in 1917. But this was research in progress as the war came to a close. In the fall of 1918, 5,000 units of one such serum reached AEF hospitals, of which 2,500 units had been used on gangrenous patients at the time of the Armistice. But there is no record of the army's trial.[10]

Even today, when physicians treating gas gangrene draw on a therapeutic arsenal that includes surgical debridement of dead and dying tissue, antibiotics, and hyperbaric oxygen therapy, the condition remains fatal for a certain number of its victims. It continues to surprise physicians "by its unexpected evolution that delays diagnosis and compromises the prognosis."[11] Today, as in the First World War, treatment can be a race against time.

Gas gangrene inevitably reached the nurses of World War I through their senses—the purplish skin or darkened muscle they saw; the bubbling and crackling sounds they heard; and above all the overpowering stench that suffused their noses, mouths, and throats and lingered with them throughout the day. Taken singly, much less together, they foretold impending death, so that sensory perception, amplified by prognostic meaning, took on the character of sensory overload. The sight or sound or scent of gas gangrene signaled that even the most intensive and inventive nursing would often come to naught. It often meant there was not much hope of survival, that the patient, "as a rule, dies pretty soon."[12] Soldiers whose strong constitutions enable them to live with the "awful poison" for an extended period simply wasted away before nurses' eyes.[13]

The scent especially overpowered nurses and threatened the steadfastness of their calling. For newly arrived nurses and volunteers, gas gangrene proved an ordeal by scent. The novelist Marie Van Horst, a New York socialite whose father, Joseph Van Horst, was a superior court judge and president of the exclusive Century Club, was living in France and writing novels when war erupted in August 1914. She lost no time in putting her Red Cross training to use and volunteering her services to the American Hospital in Paris. There she became a ward of no less than Mrs. William Vanderbilt, a patron and board member of the hospital. Shortly after Van Horst's arrival, Mrs. Vanderbilt had her assigned to the gangrene ward:

> As I went into that ward and shut the door behind me, my heart would have sunk if it had had time, but it never did. The odour seemed a conglomeration of every foul and evil thing—penetrating, dank; and from then on that terrible odour seemed to penetrate to my very bones, and when I went out into the streets of Paris I wondered what had happened to the city. When I got home I dropped my garments in an anteroom. Fancy living in that, day after day, as those nurses do; and you never get used to it—never![14]

Nurses dreaded removing original aid station bandaging, often four or five days old, because they knew they would often find the "hideous and hopeless color of gangrene."[15] The discovery of gangrene was emotionally fraught, and the gateway to its emotional power was the nose. "One feels the horrible smell in one's throat and nose all the time," wrote Edith Appleton. Marie Van Horst wrote home that she would "never forget the courage it took to take the safety-pins out of a gangrened wound for the first time."[16] The scent overwhelmed and nauseated, but vigilance was the order of the day. Nurses assigned wards of surgical cases were always alert to the postoperative appearance of gas gangrene and hemorrhage.[17] The repulsiveness of the sight and scent of gas gangrene suffused entire wards and never went away but could still be subordinated to the nurse's calling. The nurses did what they had to, but for many it remained a struggle. Among gangrene patients who survived, even changing the dressings twice a day was an "agonizing procedure."[18]

What could be done for soldiers bloated and stinking with gas gangrene? Was there any possibility of remediation? In base hospitals, specialization extended to ward care, and the gangrene cases often had a ward of their own.[19] But did it matter? Depending on the extent of infection and the promptness with which soldiers were removed to a casualty clearing station (CCS), treatment with the Carrel-Dakin method could be initiated by surgeons. Failing that, amputation of the infected limb and antiseptic irrigation, might save a soldier's life. But Carrel-Dakin's effectiveness was limited to circumscribed gangrenous sores, even deep ones that extended down to the bone.[20] It was of little use once the bacteria had spread to connective tissue, fascia, and, finally, internal organs. If exposed organs were visibly gangrenous, surgical excision could be attempted, but it was usually unsuccessful. Organ involvement suggested the infection had already spread, and the chance of surgical removal of infection from surrounding soft and connective tissue was not great.

Gangrenous organs were always a bad sign and, unless localized to a sore or small wound, made for a bleak prognosis. This was especially true for wounded soldiers left unattended in trenches and on battlefields for up to five days. By the time they received medical attention, the bacteria had not only destroyed tissue but entered the blood stream. Such blood poisoning (then termed pyemia, now septicemia) was the ne plus ultra of bacterial diffusion throughout the body. Its presence in a soldier meant immediate transfer to the moribund tent, where he awaited an agonizing death that could occur within hours, at most within days.

Among the multitude of stressors that made up ward nursing in CCSs and field hospitals, ministering to soldiers dying from gas gangrene was among the hardest to bear. What is remarkable is that even here, among the sights and sounds and smells of death, nurses occasionally rejected the medical verdict and resolved to nurse on with those awaiting death. The British sister Kate Luard provides one such example. In the midst of the Battle of Arras in May 1917, she fought on for soldiers for whom, the surgeons determined, the battle for survival was already lost. Or was it? In letters home, Luard admitted she was "engaged in a losing battle with gas gangrene again—in the Moribund Tent—a particularly fine man, too." This gangrenous patient no doubt died, but then, a month later, Luard began working with "two given-up boys" who could not be revived the preceding day. Yet to her the boys seemed "not hopeless" and she resolved to "work" on them. Here the result justified her effort, "and after more resuscitation they are now both comfortably bedded in one of the Acute Surgicals, each with a leg off and a fair chance of recovery." A few days later, she wrote that her "two resuscitated boys in the Moribund Ward are all right." Luard's feats of resuscitation did not go unnoticed; a surgeon with whom she worked remarked on his "great faith in what he calls my stunts in X Ward for them to be 'returned to stock.'"[21]

Sadly, many dying soldiers were given surgery only to develop gangrenous infections on their stumps, necessitating another surgery. Even with re-amputation followed by Carrel-Dakin irrigation, however, most would eventually die, sooner rather than later. But Luard never stopped trying. If one of her gangrenous boys was "going wrong" on a particular day, she could counter that "moribund head cases are smoking pipes and eating eggs and bread and butter. The kidney man is being dressed with [the antiseptic] Flavine and has had a leg off and is nearly convalescent!"[22] With severe gangrene cases, especially, nursing care, even if reduced to the nurse's humane caring, persisted in the face of defeat. Instances of compassion to the dying, however common on and off the battlefield, tend to be lost to history, even the intimate history captured in diaries and letters home. But there are fleeting exceptions. In March 1916 Kate Norman Derr, serving in a French Army Hospital prior to America's entry into the war, writes of a patient's arriving at the hospital from the trenches with first-aid dressings that were five days old. Under such circumstances, gangrenous infections were typically out of control and death a certainty. And yet, Derr recalled, she reached out to the soldier, and "slipped in to do something perfectly useless that might perhaps give a ray of comfort."[23]

The vast majority of nursing saves went unrecorded, noticed at the time by a colleague, a supervisor, perhaps even the head matron. Without the wartime diaries and letters the nurses left behind, we would have little inkling of their quiet struggles to keep the medically forsaken alive. Their struggles take us far from the world of high-tech nursing, even in its low-tech World War I incarnation. What we behold, again and again, is hard-core, soft-touch nursing, abetted by a Rube Goldberg inventiveness in making use of materials at hand, somehow garnering materials not obtainable, and then patiently titrating treatments (including food intake) in a manner responsive to states of severe, even deathlike, debilitation.

> A little night sister in the Medical last night pulled a man round who was at the point of death, in the most splendid way. He had bronchitis and acute Bright's Disease, and Captain S. and the day sister had all but given him up; but at 10:30 p.m., as a last resource, Captain S. talked about a Vapour Bath [steaming up his room], and the little sister got hold of a Primus [stove] and some tubing and a kettle and cradles, and got it going, and did it again later, and this morning the man was speaking and swallowing, and back to earth again. He is still alive tonight, but not much more.[24]

The nurses' diaries and letters record other instances of heroic nursing in the face of grievous wounds and medical resignation. On occasion, nursing interventions save soldiers long enough to persuade surgeons to operate on those they had earlier passed over. Two such examples come to us from Kate Norman Derr and Kate Luard, respectively:

> You will like to hear of the living skeleton with wounds in back and hands and shoulder that they brought me filthy and nearly dead from another pavilion. That was nine days ago. I diagnosed him as a case of neglect and slow starvation, and treated him accordingly—malted milk, eggs, soap, and alcohol to the fore. His dressing took one and a half hours every day, and all nourishment given a few drops at a time, and early all the time, for he was almost too weak to lift an eyelid, much less a finger. This morning he actually laughed with me and tried to clench his fist inside the dressings to show me how strong he was. He's *saved*, and that makes up for much.[25]

> I happened on a corpse-like child [a teenage soldier] the other day being brought into the Moribund Ward to die and we got to work on resuscitation, with some success. He had been bleeding from his subclavian artery and heard them leave him for dead in his shell-hole. But he crawled out and was eventually tended in a dug-out by "a lad what said prayers with me," and later the hole in his chest was plugged and he reached us—what was left of him. When, after two days, he belonged to this world again, I got Capt. B. to see him, and he got Major C. to operate and tied the twisted artery which I had re-plugged—he couldn't be touched before—and cover with muscle the hole through which he was breathing, and he is now a great hero known as "the Prince of Wales."[26]

• • •

"We have horribly bad wounds in numbers—some crawling with maggots, some stink and tense with gangrene." This is the British nursing sister Edith Appleton, working out of General Hospital No. 1 in Étretat in July 1916.[27] The pairing of wounds infested with maggots and wounds reeking of gangrene is not surprising. Both repulsed the nurses, and both required steely resolve in order to nurse on. It is human nature to be repelled by the repellant. How not to believe, as Beatrice Hopkinson did, that a soldier's "terrible state" had something to do with the maggot-filled wounds that surgeons laid bare on the operating table?[28] Their initial reaction to insect invaders was instinctive and gendered, if not in the strong sense of their Civil War predecessors, for whom womanly sensibility, confronted with thin, slimy maggots, threatened to overwhelm nursing duty altogether.[29]

The irony of the pairing is that whereas stink of gas gangrene signified life-threatening infection, the sight of maggots signified life. Hopkinson's patient died two days following his surgery because, by the time he reached the operating table, he had spent several days lying in no man's land with an infected double fracture of the tibia. The maggots did not hasten his demise; they exerted themselves to forestall it. For maggots were actually healing allies, a gift of nature, so to speak. Nor did their ability to clean out infected tissue and promote healing await World War I. Ambroise Paré observed the healing effect of fly larvae on wounds during the Battle of Saint-Quentin of 1557, and Baron Dominique-Jean Larrey, Napoleon's surgeon-in-chief, reported on the accelerated growth of new tissue (granulation) and shortened healing time of maggot-infested wounded in 1829. During the American Civil War, J. F. Zacharias, an assistant surgeon with the Army of Tennessee, took the next step: He applied maggot larvae to infected wounds to promote healing.

The orderlies, nurses, and surgeons of the Western front repeated these observations a half century later. They noticed that, especially among wounded soldiers left on the battlefield for several days, wounds infested with maggots were cleaner and healed faster than those that were maggot-free. The reason, simply, is that maggots only feed on dead and dying human tissue. And while consuming it, they excrete a chemical cocktail—ammonia, urea, allantoin, calcium carbonate, specific cytokines [proteins]—that stimulates tissue regeneration (i.e., granulation) in wounds they have cleaned out.[30]

So the nurses of the Great War learned to welcome their instinctive revulsion at the sight of slimy, wormlike insects crawling around under filthy bandages. Maggots might remain "horrifying creatures," but in their benignity, they simultaneously became "strange little organisms" whose healing power was gratefully acknowledged. These are the words of the American nurse Shirley Millard, who in March 1918 joined a contingent of volunteer nurses at a French evacuation hospital at Chateau in northcentral France. In July, she observed the massive stomach wound of a young soldier from Nebraska:

> In the huge wound was a seething mass of living writhing insects. I weakened for a moment. I thought I knew just about everything, but I had never seen this before. I beckoned to an orderly. He came and took one look.
> "Maggots," he said. "I'll get you a can of ether. That kills them." At first I thought I couldn't do it, but I did. The orderly explained that this was a natural, even a healthy symptom. I watched the squirming mass wither and die under the ether. When I removed them I saw that the wound was clean and fresh. These strange little organisms, it appears, eat away the decay and prevent infection of the blood stream. I soon learned to welcome the uncovering of these horrifying creatures, for often the removal of bandages revealed the hideous and hopeless color of gangrene.[31]

The observations of maggot-accelerated wound healing on the battlefields of the Western front came to fruition after the war. Among those who observed the effects of maggots on battlefield wounds was William Baer, an orthopedic surgeon from John Hopkins Medical College. After the war, Baer returned to Hopkins and in the late 1920s began systematically applying maggot larvae to non-healing soft tissue wounds at Johns Hopkins Hospital. His findings bore out his wartime observations and led to mainstream acceptance of maggot debridement therapy (MDT) beginning in 1931, the year Baer published his report on the successful treatment of four children with chronic osteomyelitis (bone infection) with maggots.[32] Through the end of World War II, MDT was used in over 300 hospitals in the United States alone. With the availability of antibiotics after the war, however, it fell into disuse for almost half a century, only to return in the 1990s, when new strains of antibiotic-resistant bacteria summoned the uncelebrated larvae of the green bottle fly back to the war against infection. The larvae are now raised under sterile conditions in laboratories whence, as "medicinal maggots," they are shipped to hospitals and wound centers worldwide. MDT is now an accepted alternative treatment for chronic soft tissue infections—whether caused by abscesses, burns, ulcers, cellulitis, or gangrene—that prove resistant to drug therapy. Contemporary physicians and nurses, some of whom are still deterred by the "yuck" factor,[33] have relearned the empirical finding of nurses and orderlies who beheld clean wounds beneath masses of maggots when they unbandaged wounded soldiers brought to them off the battlefields of the Western front.[34]

• • •

Infected fractures, especially of the femur or thigh bone, were another dreaded complication of delayed evacuation of the wounded from the battlefield. The risk of gas gangrene for neglected thigh fractures was especially high. Complicated fractures also followed from grenade and gunshot wounds to the lower extremities suffered in marshes and during heavy rains. Fortunately, a promising new method for treatment of extreme wound-related fractures had been developed just three years before the outbreak of war in Europe, and it too placed new demands on war nurses at the front. The Balkan frame (or Balkan beam) comprised single or double longitudinal metal beams placed above a hospital bed and permitted fractured arms and legs, especially fractures of the femur, to be suspended in traction in a semi-flexed position. Its inventor, the Croatian surgeon Vatroslav Florschütz, devised the apparatus at the civil hospital of Osijek (Croatia) in 1911. Word of the invention traveled quickly, and it was used in the Serbian-Bulgarian War of 1913, where its benefits were immediately apparent.[35] But the device came into its own in the fracture wards of World War I, where both sides employed it on a routine basis. On the Russian and Western fronts alike, nurses became adepts in its use, virtuoso adjusters of the heavy weights and cables that maintained constant traction of fractured long bones suspended from the overhead beam. At *L'Hôpital Jacobean*, the American nurse Mary Gray ran the ward for compound fractures that utilized both Balkan frames and newly developed fracture reduction apparatus.[36]

An alternative approach to stabilizing compound long bone fractures was Buck's extension, an early type of skin traction that preserved limb length and reduced pain while the casted fracture healed. It was developed by the Civil War surgeon Gordon Buck in 1877, and came into use in the 1880s, when civilian surgeons employed it not only for long bone fractures but for spine and joint injuries as well.[37] It may have found very occasional use in the Spanish-American and

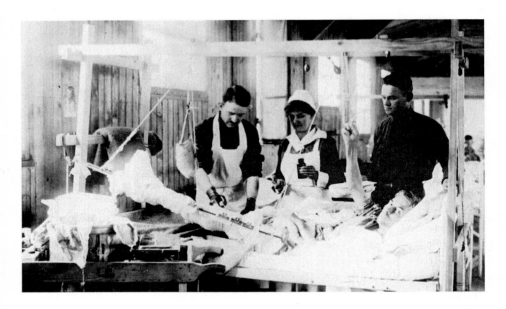

World War I surgeon, nurse, and orderly at the bedside of a soldier whose leg is suspended from a Balkan frame (Library of Congress).

Boer Wars at century's end, but there is no specific mention of its use by the American or British military. In both conflicts, battlefield injuries of any type were dwarfed by infectious disease—typhoid, yellow fever, dysentery, malaria—and nursing revolved around bed care of the stricken. Like other treatment methods devised in the late-nineteenth and early-twentieth century, Buck's extension only came into its own in the hands of the nurses of the Great War. Along with the Balkan frame, it remains a mainstay of modern orthopedics, and its operation, then and now, is simple. If, for example, a patient has fractured his right tibia, then his leg is kept straight by a cord attached to an extension off his right foot. The cord is attached to a pulley which, in turn, is attached to a weight in front of the bed. The foot of the bed is often elevated to provide counter-traction that keeps the patient from being pulled toward the foot of the bed.

The prevalence of compound fractures of the thigh bone during the war meant that Buck's extension (aka Buck's skin traction), no less than the Balkan frame, came under the purview of nurses, especially those assigned to fracture wards. It was yet another device in their procedural arsenal. And they were expected not only to know how to use it, but to understand why exactly it was being used. Today, Buck's extension is made of newer materials and has an even broader range of application (e.g., for hip fractures and lower back pain), but the device is very much what it was during the Great War, and Elizabeth Bundy's description of it in her textbook of 1917 for American military nurses has a contemporary ring. Buck's extension apparatus, she begins, "is or should be familiar to every nurse who will have occasion to apply it frequently in caring for surgical cases in military hospitals." After briefly explaining the principle of the device, she proceeds to its set up:

> To the part below the injury a wide strip of adhesive plaster is securely applied on either side, extending well below the extremity of the limb. To these strips a weight is attached by means of a cord and pulley, with an intervening foot piece, which will keep the part at rest. Counter-extension is secured by some device which pulls the upper fragment of bone in the opposite direction. For

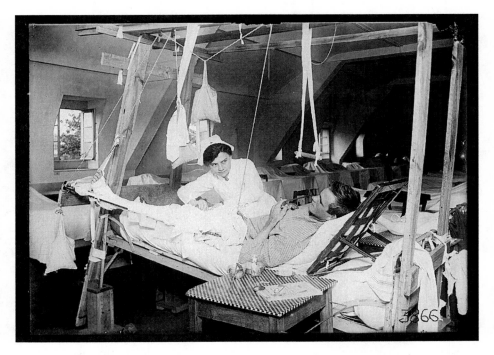

An American nurse tends a wounded soldier in multiple traction devices, including Buck's extension, in Évreux, France, in 1918. She is performing small adjustments to help him find the a more comfortable leg position (Library of Congress).

example, when a lower extremity in extension is elevated and the foot of the bed as well, the weight of the body inclining toward the head of the bed furnishes a means of counter-extension.[38]

Setting up Buck's extension was not a once-and-for-all affair. The apparatus required ongoing monitoring and adjustment to function properly. In the years leading up to the war, when nursing care for patients with major fractures took place in the home, the adjusting of traction apparatuses was a major order of business for trained nurses. Writing in the *American Journal of Nursing* in 1908, Marion Parsons, a graduate of Boston City Hospital Training School and operating room nurse in Boston's Boothby Surgical Hospital, made plain that nurses alone bore responsibility for the outcome of treatment. In the case of Buck's extension, Nurse Parsons offered cautions aplenty. Nurses were enjoined to attend diligently to the following:

> [T]he sole of the foot must not rest against the foot of the bed because of loss of extension; the T-splint must not become loose and slip up or down or twist to one side; the straps holding the coaptation splints must be kept tight. It should be borne in mind that any displacement of the apparatus for holding the leg will allow corresponding displacement of the fragments of bone and cause delayed union and shortening of the limb. Whatever apparatus is used, the nurse should fully understand what it is meant to accomplish, that she may keep it working properly.[39]

It was an exacting business, to which the nurse's responsibility for finding an appropriate bed in the home (e.g., one without a solid foot-board) or modifying the patient's own bed to accommodate the device was added. But it helped prepare American nurses for wartime service, when use of the Balkan frame and proper adjustment of Buck's extension and other traction devices were at the center of daily management of long-bone fractures. Whereas Buck's extension was the traction of choice for fractures of the lower leg, Blake's extension, which stabilized the leg from above, with the pulley and weight extending down the head of the bed, was often the traction of choice for fractures of the thigh bone (femur). But none of the traction devices eliminated the need for orthopedic ingenuity when it was called for. Using materials at hand, nurses devised their own solutions for musculoskeletal injuries in an effort to restore limb function. Kate Norman Derr once again provides an example of such ingenuity in action. She wrote home from Vitry in April 1917 of a soldier with badly damaged knee joints and of her "lastingly satisfactory" work on this soldier with "double anthrotomie [deep lacerations] of the knees." She explained that

> when he came the insteps were bent like a ballet-dancer's. Even admitting his recovery, which seemed impossible, he would be obliged to go about on the points of his toes, the knees being permanently stiff. At first, after "peeling" with every conceivable dissolvent, I began just the slightest *effleurissage* [circular stroking] which developed into massage, and then I invented an apparatus.... A board about 14 inches square was padded with cotton and swathed neatly in a bandage. This was laid vertical against the soles of the feet which I tried to place as nearly as possible in a normal position. Then I attached a bandage (having no elastic, which would have been better) to the head rail of the bed on one side, passed it around the board and up the other side, fastening it again to the rail as taut as possible. The knot was tightened twice a day. Result—in two weeks those refractory feet had regained a proper attitude.[40]

Not to be outdone, Grace Gassette, a coworker of Alexis Carrel who superintended the surgical dressing room at the American

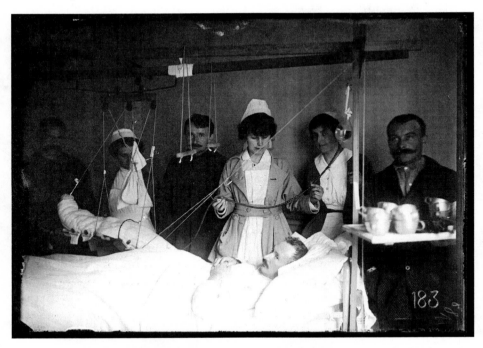

Nurses inspect a patient's multiple traction devices, one of which is Blake's extension for upper thigh fracture, at Dr. Blake's Hospital, Paris, 1918 (Library of Congress).

Hospital in Neuilly for two years, invented over 60 simple but effective orthopedic devices that enabled fractured limbs to remain firmly in place while permitting wounds to drain. Untold amputations were prevented through use of the devices, and by November 1917, Gassette and her hospital coworkers had supplied 50 military hospitals with 6,000 of these various appliances. "You will pass the rest of your life as an orthopedic consultant," a surgeon consulting for the American government told her. The French government recognized her contributions in a more concrete manner: It made her a Chevalier of the Legion of Honor. Still, Gassette found time to harness her inventiveness on behalf of orthopedic patients with special needs. For a soldier with two fractured vertebrae, for example, whose plaster cast prevented him from walking, she designed and constructed a well-padded aluminum corset. "The first day he wore it," she recounted, "he walked about normally, as happy as a child."[41]

Total care, in times of war or peace, can only mean totally individualized care. In World War I, it also means dedication to severely injured individuals in the face of bombings that reached and occasionally destroyed the clearing stations and field hospitals where the nurses labored. In Belgium in the fall of 1917, enemy bombs destroyed the 58th General Scottish Hospital adjacent to Beatrice Hopkinson's own 59th. Hopkinson watched while orderlies from her hospital "stooped over bunches of twigs in various places and picked up something, putting it in the sheet. They were the arms and legs and other pieces of the patients that had been bombed and blown right out into the [outlying] park."[42] Now the U.S. Army has Mortuary Affairs specialists who retrieve and bag body parts and liquefied innards of fallen soldiers in Afghanistan.[43] In World War I, the army medical corps had orderlies with sheets. Back in her own hospital, with bombs continuing to rain down, Hopkinson confided to her diary that "My knees just shook and, had I allowed it, my teeth would have rattled; but I had to be brave for my patients' sake. When they saw the womenfolk apparently without fear it kept them brave."[44] To sequester fear without projecting it into others has been the gift of battlefield nurses of all wars. To remain calmly on task when the very infrastructure that supports nursing is at risk—this capacity, perhaps, is her or his true measure. It draws on other instruments in the nurse's palliative arsenal, one of which is an instrument of traditional nursing care on which the battlefield places heightened demands.

• • •

The nurses of the Great War had their hands. In reception huts their hands were instruments of differential diagnosis that were essential to the triaging process. Mary Borden provides a powerful rendering of the role of hands in the reception hut of her Belgian CCS. "It was my nursing business," she begins,

> to sort out the wounded as they were brought in from the ambulances and to keep them from dying before they got to the operating rooms: it was my business to sort out the nearly dying from the dying. I was there to sort them out and tell how fast life was ebbing in them. Life was leaking away in all of them; but with some there was no hurry, with others it was a case of minutes.... My hand could tell of itself one kind of cold from another. They were all half-frozen when they arrived, but the chill of their icy flesh wasn't the same as the cold inside them when life was almost ebbed away. My hands could instantly tell the difference between the cold of the harsh bitter night and the stealthy cold of death. Then there was another thing, a small fluttering thing. I didn't think about it or count it. My fingers felt it. I was in a dream, led this way and that by my cute eyes and hands that did many things, and, seemed to know what to do.[45]

The role of hands in determining when soldiers were fighting for life and when relinquishing the struggle was no doubt greatest in reception huts such as Borden's. But it extended to the wards as well. A hand that closed around the nurse's hand less tightly than previously did not augur well, whereas a previously enfeebled hand that held the nurse's tightly was an encouraging sign.[46]

Nursing hands were also instruments of treatment when injuries did not require the surgeon's attention; they debrided wounds, dug out shrapnel and high-explosive shell fragments, and dressed and bandaged them. Nursing hands adjusted Carrel-Dakin apparatus, Balkan frames, and Buck's and Blake's extensions; they also devised a variety of orthopedic aids for fracture management and wound drainage. Hands betrayed the strain of nurses laboring on in exhaustion, and hands conveyed the gratitude of injured soldiers for nursing ministrations that meant the difference between sleepless pain and restful sleep.

It is December 1914. As she finished up her 12-hour shift and prepares to leave the American Hospital in Neuilly, Marie von Horst bids the nine men in her ward good night. She notices that the ward's latest arrival, an ordinary soldier, is sitting upright "with an appealing expression on his pale, agreeable face." She asks, with some trepidation, whether she can do anything for him. He meekly remarks that his back injuries have prevented him from sleeping for two nights and wonders whether she might take a look at his wounds. Van Horst is a newly arrived Red Cross volunteer and realizes that what she finds underneath the bandages may be more than she can deal with on her own. So she searches for one of the sisters but, finding none at hand, feels she must comply with her patient's request and do what she can. So she unbandages him and finds

> across his back two wounds, whose width and whose gaping mouths cried to Heaven. I think it took me about half an hour to wash them, to cleanse them and bind him up again. By that time my hands were trembling and my limbs were almost beyond my own control.[47]

It is van Horst who then has a sleepless night, wondering what will happen to her patient if she failed to do her work well, if through

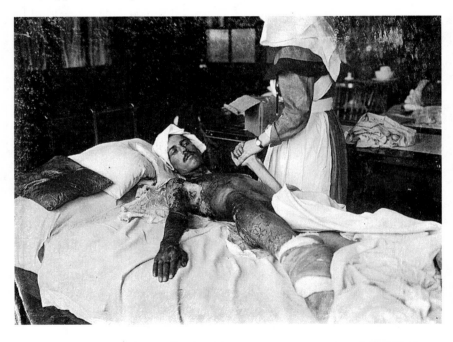

A Red Cross nurse holds the hand of Sergeant Sawyer Spence, severely burned by poison gas, Nottingham Hospital, England (copyright © Jon Spence and reprinted with permission).

carelessness she "had infected those pitiful slits." Tired and miserable, she returns to the ward early the next morning only to find her patient sitting up in bed, "his cheeks quite pink. He held out one of his hands to me as I crossed the floor. Merci, merci, ma soeur, I slept all night as I used to sleep when I was a boy and did not know what war was."[48] So van Horst has passed the test, her patient's joyfully extended hand redeeming the work of her uncertain, trembling hands.

Nursing hands also monitor the nurse's own performance, especially the acclimatization of new nurses to the demands of the reception hut. Shirley Millard reports how her hands "get firmer, faster. I can feel the hardness of emergency setting in. Perhaps after a while I won't mind."[49] More importantly, nursing hands stabilize soldiers whose fear and pain off the battlefield leave them overwhelmed and childlike. With soldiers who arrive at casualty clearing stations in surgical shock, massive blood loss is compounded by sepsis, pain, and anxiety, making it incumbent on nurses not only to institute stabilizing measures, but to make the soldier feel "he is in good and safe hands."[50] Touch is a potent instrument for inducing this feeling. Soldiers clutch hands as they ask, "Is it all right? Don't leave me."[51] But it is usually not all right, and it is the nurse's hand that provides a lifeline of human attachment to relieve a desolation that is often wordless: "Reaching down to feel his legs before I could stop him, he uttered a heartbreaking scream. I held his hand firmly until the drug I had given him took effect." When panic overwhelms and leaves soldiers mute, the hand communicates what the voice cannot: "He seized my hand and gripped it until it hurt…. He looked up at me desperately, hanging onto my hand in his panic." The hand offers consolation when there are no words: "The bandage around his eyes was soaked with tears. I sat on his bed and covered his hand with mine."[52]

The nurse's hands mark attachment and impending loss. Soldiers become terrified at the time of surgery. The reality of amputation, the painful aftercare it will entail, and the kind of life it permits thereafter can be overwhelming. It is 1915, and the American Maud Mortimer is in a field hospital at the edge of Belgium, only five miles from the firing line. A patient with whom she has connected, "Petit Pere," is about to have his leg amputated. He makes her promise that when he comes around from the anesthesia she will be there, and that she will "hold his hand through the first most painful dressing." The amputation complete, he gazes up at her: "Hold my hand tight and I will scream no more."[53]

But the attachment can transcend treatment-related trauma and become perduring. Now it is April 1918, three years later, and a pause in the action permits Helen Boylston's hospital to ship 26 ward patients to England. One of her patients, Hilley, begs her to let him remain. "I went out to the ambulance with him," she recounts, "and he clung tightly to my hand all the way. I almost cried."[54] Such separation, with the hand clinging it elicits, reminds us that a wounded soldier's parting from his nurses can be a major loss, even when it is a prelude to greater safety and fuller recovery. The vigorous hand clinging of the living, even in loss, is far preferable to the enfeebled squeeze of the dying. With the latter, the nurse 's hand becomes an instrument of palliation, interposing human touch between living and dying, easing the transition from one to the other: "I held his hand as he went.... Near the end he saw me crying and patted my hand with his two living fingers to comfort me."[55] Expressions of gratitude and affection, hand-communicated, are part of the process. The hand continues to communicate as the body shuts down: "He was ever so good and tried to take milk and food almost up to the end but he was unable to speak and not really conscious, though he could hold my hand and squeeze it which was so sweet of him."[56]

The use of the hand as an amplifier of treatment, a spur to recovery, a tactile communiqué that the soldier's wounds, however grave, are now *in* hand; the use of the hand as a vehicle of comfort care when treatment fails and death is *at* hand—these aspects of human touch hardly originate on the Western front. In the Spanish-American War, Sister X recalls, head injuries were the most distressing of all, since they often left soldiers paralyzed and also without speech or hearing. One such soldier appears to her "in a great state of mind," clutching at her hand as he tries to speak and "gazing at me in an agonized way."[57] The Red Cross nurse Alice Bron, walking back to her hospital near Jacobsdal in the first year of the Boer War, is summoned by soldiers to a dying comrade. She sees at once that death is at hand:

> Introducing a spatula between his teeth, I separated the clenched jaws, and administered a few drops of whisky; then I wiped his face with my apron and asked him how he felt. The sense of hearing, I have observed, exists until the last, and I advise nurses to speak to the dying, encourage them, and promise

them a speedy recovery—a white lie for which there is no cause to blush. As he did not appear to hear me, I took his hands in mine. His fingers contracted feebly, like those of a little, little child, on mine, as if to hold them.

"My poor fellow, you will soon be better," I said.[58]

Civil War nurses who ventured onto the battlefield or labored in tented field hospitals knew all too well the role of hands as instruments of containment in the face of intolerable suffering and impending death. For patients in extremis, whether physically or mentally or both, the nurse's hand provided what the psychoanalyst Donald Winnicott termed a "holding environment."[59] "Scenes of fresh horror rose up before us each day. Tales of suffering were told, which elsewhere would have well-nigh frozen the blood with horror. We grew callous to the sight of blood, and great gashed lips opened under our untrembling hands, while from there [*sic*] ruggedness slowly dripped the life of the victim." This is the Union nurse Sophronia Bucklin from the amputation tent of a field hospital in northern Virginia in 1863.[60]

The reaching out with hands, the holding of and being held by hands, is bidirectional. A nurse reaches out for a patient's hand and takes it in her own. A patient reaches out for a nurse's hand and either clutches it firmly or holds it weakly or pats it gratefully. A dying patient "bade me good-by so touchingly, holding my hand in his poor trembling ones." This is the Union nurse Emily Parsons from Benton Barracks Hospital, St. Louis in April 1863.[61] She knows the men are beginning to care for her, she writes her mother, because "as I stop at the beds as I go round, the hands are put out to take mine, and I must hear how they are, and say something to them." She writes further of how and when hands are extended to her: "There is something that goes to your heart in those rough, worn hands, that have carried their guns through many a hard fight for our country, and are right ready to carry them again."[62]

As the sick and wounded arrive at Parsons' hospital in early July 1863 following the battles of Vicksburg and Milliken's Bend, Parsons writes her mother of "how touching it is to see the soldiers watch for a greeting and a touch of the hand." The soldiers, she adds, "are very shy of claiming notice." Each lies gravely on his bed until she addresses him, and then "the whole face lights up and the rough worn hands are held out."[63]

The convergence of caregiving, touching, and being touched, a legacy especially of the nursing care of the Crimean War and the

Civil War, remains part of the nurse's professional identity even today, when much hands-on care is relegated to practical nurses and nurse aides. This is one reason that contemporary nursing literature is more nuanced than medical literature on the phenomenology and dynamic meanings of touch. Nursing research, for example, has parsed the tactile components of touch—duration, location, intensity, and sensation—and also differentiated between comfort (i.e., expressive) touch and procedural (i.e., instrumental) touch, the latter being the touch associated with performing procedures.[64]

Among nurses, expressive touch and procedural touch have different historical timelines. Whereas a professional ethos that privileged patient care emerged during the Crimean War and blossomed during the Civil War, this ethos, with rare exceptions, pertained to expressive touch. This is because mid-nineteenth-century military medicine, in its nonsurgical procedural aspects, was in its infancy. There was simply less to do of a procedural nature outside the operating tent, and very little, other than dressing and bandaging wounds, that surgeons could relegate to nurses. Here again, the Great War is the fulcrum that propelled nurses toward modern nursing practice, since by 1914 the laying on of hands was linked to procedural interventions unavailable in previous wars.

We have briefly surveyed the range of these procedures and the contexts in which they occurred: in reception huts, where nurses controlled massive bleeds, stabilized soldiers in shock, removed accessible shrapnel, and splinted fractured limbs; in surgical tents, where nurses administered general anesthesia and assisted in operations; and in wards, where nurses routinely chose medications to manage pain and control infection, performed minor bedside surgeries, and monitored deep wound irrigation, especially via the Carrel-Dakin method. In these and other ways, the nurses' hands joined those of the surgeons as tools of treatment that usually eased suffering and often saved lives. Whereas the expressive touch of Civil War nurses was bolstered by their status as surrogate mothers and Christian guarantors of a beneficent afterlife,[65] the expressive touch of Great War nurses was heightened by the procedural touch that rendered their hands, both to their patients and to themselves, instruments of scientific healing. The hands extended to wounded and dying soldiers were not only—and, in most cases, not primarily—the hands of caring mothers (or sisters or spouses) but of nursing professionals who, caught in the bloody wreckage of total war, embraced an ethos of total care.

◆ ◆ ◆

Nurses such as Beatrice Hopkinson, Agnes Warner, Helen Boylston, Kate Luard, Shirley Millard, Edith Appleton, and Kate Norman Derr did not see themselves as brave. Rather, their sense of duty was powerful enough to sequester fear and compel action in ways that would have been all but incomprehensible to their non-nursing selves. The transition to battlefield nursing called on nurses to block out the wounded soldier's relational world, to cultivate what the American psychiatrist Harry Stack Sullivan, lecturing in the aftermath of the Second World War, termed "selective inattention."[66] This was formalized in the advice given to nurses headed overseas. "The wounds which you will be called on to handle and dress are such that you have never imagined it possible for a human being to be so fearfully hurt and yet to be alive," cautioned Alice Fitzgerald in an article expressly for these nurses in the December 1917 issue of the *American Journal of Nursing.* "If the man is seriously crippled or disfigured, it will be well to try not to think too much of his wife, of his children, or his parents, who are anxiously waiting for news of him 'over there.'"[67]

To be sure, not all nurses were up to the rigors of battlefield nursing, but those who proved (euphemistically) "inefficient" or otherwise unable to function were "quickly weeded out."[68] The vast majority stepped into their new roles, and once at work in CCSs and the wards of field and base hospitals, it did not take long for Fitzgerald's strategies of self-protection to become automatic as new nurses embraced, consciously and pridefully, an overarching sense of duty. "I never realized what the word 'duty' meant until this War," Beatrice Hopkinson remarked. Hers was the courage of the Hippocratic caregiver, who subordinates all self-interest to the patient's well-being. For the American nurses of the First World War, no less than for their compatriots from other nations, such subordination extended to self-preservation itself. Those who wrote about night time bombing raids, with enemy artillery batteries "banging away and shaking the whole hut with vibrations," managed to bracket their own anxiety. They became able to record the destruction while channeling their concern onto their patients, especially those who were shell shocked.[69] Occasionally, as we shall see, nurses too were shocked into dysfunction.

I admire the nurses because their sense of mission remained unswerving as moribund wards swelled, and they failed time and again to "pull round" those wounded too far gone to be pulled. Living and working amid the bodies of those they failed to save—perhaps *because* they lived and worked among those they failed—the nurses remained certain of who they were and why they endured what they did. They were vindicated by their calling, and the calling empowered them.

And with the resolve to nurse on, even during bombing raids that imperiled them, came defiant resiliency. The clearing stations right off the front were, in the words of American nurse and poet Mary Borden, the second battlefield. It was a battlefield littered with the weapons of nursing care—caregiving paraphernalia that combatted and succumbed to the inexorability of death. Borden was not alone in making the analogy. "The wards are like battlefields," remarked Kate Luard during the battle of Arras in April 1917, "with battered wrecks in every bed and on stretchers between the beds and down the middles." Her simile captures both the chaotic totality and the individualized terror and agony of those who formed the wreckage. The New York socialite and Red Cross volunteer Marie Van Horst beheld a severely wounded soldier screaming terribly as the doctor dresses his wounds. A very young soldier, a "Welsh boy," leaned over and handed her his glass of lemonade, hoping she will give it to his comrade. Perhaps it would ease his torment a bit and quiet his inconsolable wails. "He could not bear those cries," Van Horst tells us. "They were worse than the battle."[70]

So why did the nurses labor on? Many nurses were taken to the brink of desolation but, with few recorded exceptions—and despite the impact of their self-questioning epiphanies—they resisted falling over the edge. The fact is that by 1914, military medical and nursing care was modern, and it allowed the nursing ethos to bear fruit. "He's *saved*, and that makes up for much," declaimed Kate Norman Derr in the fall of 1915. To which Kate Luard added her own gloss a year and a half later:

> Some of us and Capt. B. have been having a bad fit of pessimism over them all lately, wondering what is the good of operations, nursing, rescues, or anything, when so many have died in the end. But even a few miraculous recoveries buck one up to begin again.[71]

4

Poison Gas

"Mustard gas burns. Terrific suffering."[1]

Chemical warfare, sad to say, spans the ancient and modern worlds. Arrows and spears tipped with poison (e.g., snake venom) were supposedly used during the Trojan War of 1185 B.C., and early Greek writings from 431 B.C. tell of the Spartans' use of burning tar pitch mixed with sulphur to produce a suffocating gas during the Peloponnesian War. At the other end of the timeline, we have Iraqi insurgents' use of chlorine in Baghdad truck bombings in 2007 and the Syrian air force's chemical attack on the rebel-held town of Khan Sheikhoun in 2017. The American Civil War was rife with civilian proposals to use various chemicals to incapacitate opposing troops. Cayenne pepper, liquid chloroform and chlorine, hydrogen cyanide, arsenic compounds, caustic acids—all to be loaded into explosive artillery shells. In the Confederacy, fume-producing chemical agents were actually prepared and demonstrated, but they were never used.[2] In the Anglo-Boer War at century's end, British forces used artillery shells filled with picric acid. On explosion they released the chemical lyddite, which caused carbon monoxide poisoning and suffocation, an unintended consequence of combustion.

Everything became intentional in World War I, which saw the first large-scale use of chemical weapons in modern industrialized warfare. German, French, and British scientists were all experimenting with tear gas by the fall of 1914, but the German army's chief of staff, Erich von Falkenhayn, sought a more potent asphyxiant that would put enemy soldiers out of action—permanently. The charge was led by the gifted German chemist Fritz Haber, whose prewar work revolved around the Haber-Bosch process, a chemical reaction that "fixed" (i.e., rendered stable as a compound) atmospheric nitrogen and hydrogen into ammonia. The result was the commercial production of nitrogen-based fertilizers that vastly increased agricultural yields and significantly eased world-wide hunger. For this work, Haber received the 1918 Nobel Prize in Chemistry.

With the outbreak of war in 1914, however, Haber, a German patriot of the first rank, subordinated his research to the war effort. Heeding the call of the German High Command, he headed the Chemistry Section of the Ministry of War, where he led the team that developed chlorine gas to drive enemy troops out of their trenches.[3] Haber himself recruited and trained the "gas troops" that, with favorable winds, would open the valves of steel cylinders filled with chlorine under high pressure. During the Second Battle of Ypres, Belgium, in April 1915, with Haber in attendance, Germany released 5,730 cylinders of chlorine gas across a four-mile stretch of no man's land into the Allied lines. This was the "cloud gas" or "drift gas" that, on first use, caused an entire French Colonial division of Algerians to flee, its soldiers literally choking to death.

Allied leaders, British Field Marshall John French among them, reacted to the first gas attack with shock and outrage. Germany's action was not only inhumane but in clear violation of The Hague Conventions and Declarations of 1899, whereby signatory nations agree not to use projectiles that released asphyxiating gases or weapons "calculated to cause unnecessary suffering."[4] But the initial outrage did not mitigate the need to respond in kind: The British released cylinders of chlorine gas during the Battle of Loos the following summer. Later that year, French chemists led by Victor Grignard developed phosgene gas, a far deadlier chemical agent whose effectiveness was increased by combining it with chlorine, since the latter's vapors helped to spread the denser phosgene. The combination was first used by the Germans against British troops at Wieltje (near Ypres) in mid–December 1915, but its devastating effectiveness was demonstrated by the Austrians, who used it to deliver a crushing blow to the Italian lines on Monte San Michele on June 29, 1916. Germany upped the horror yet again in July 1917, when it delivered artillery shells filled with dichlor-ethylsulphide or "mustard gas" just prior to the Third Battle of Ypres.

Mustard gas had been synthesized by the German chemist Victor Meyer in 1886, and its weaponization three decades later capped the collaboration of German science with the military during the war. Here, finally, was a gas that could be loaded into artillery shells as a heavy oily liquid that evaporated on explosion. Nor could its crippling effects be prevented by gas masks, since it burned through clothing, destroyed underlying skin, and caused inflammation all over the body. The moister parts of the body—faces, armpits, genitalia—were especially vulnerable.

Chlorine and phosgene gas attacked the airways. Severe respiratory swelling and inflammation killed many instantly, and the rest struggled to nearby casualty clearing stations with acute congestion of the lungs and usually temporary blindness. Phosgene, being almost odorless, tended to be inhaled more deeply and for longer periods than chlorine. Soldiers who had inhaled the most gas arrived with heavy discharge of a frothy yellow fluid from their noses and mouths as they drowned in their own secretions. For the rest, partial suffocation persisted for days, and long-term survivors often had permanent lung damage, chronic bronchitis, and occasionally heart failure.

Mustard gas, a deadly blistering agent or "vesicant," accounted for 70 percent of the 1.3 million poison gas casualties of the war.[5] It burned the skin and respiratory tract, stripping the mucous membrane off the bronchial tubes and causing inflammation of the eyes

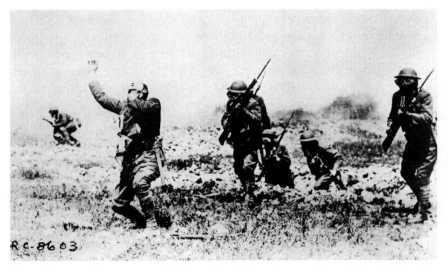

American soldiers, one of whom is without a mask and clutching his face, flee a German gas attack.

(conjunctivitis) and light sensitivity (photophobia) so extreme that eyelids remained sealed shut for days or even weeks. Off the battlefield, soldiers expectorated bloody pus, sometimes filled with dead tissue or "slough" of the tracheal and bronchial mucous membrane. The sloughing off of membrane left a septic raw surface that, after two days of simple breathing, usually developed into necrotizing bronchopneumonia—a bacterial infection of the bronchi and lungs so severe that it killed living tissue. This became the proximate cause of death.

Among those spared pneumonia, deep penetration of the gas led to internal and external bleeding over the following week. Victims were left in excruciating pain and utterly helpless; many died within a month. Convalescence for severe skin burns, major respiratory disease, and severe conjunctivitis and photophobia typically took 45–60 days. Soldiers who survived their ordeal were likely to go through life with asthma, emphysema, chronic bronchitis, and/or chronic conjunctivitis.[6] Even today, when post-exposure therapy includes laser or needle debridement, collagen-laminated nylon dressings, and anti-inflammatory agents, mustard gas wounds exact their toll. Treatment remains supportive, with serious long-term consequences of industrial exposure reported as recently as 2004.[7]

Nurses of World War I, no less than physicians, were initially confused about the nature of the gas and the severity of its effects.[8] They were quickly brought up to speed and realized that soldiers suffering from poison gas posed a nursing challenge no less formidable than those dying from gangrenous wounds. Nurses were accustomed to losing patients but not to being powerless to provide comfort care, to ease patients' agony during their final days. But how to nurse on when nursing was unavailing, when the burns were so terrible that "nothing seems to give relief," indeed, when "blinded eyes and scorched throats and blistered bodies made the struggle for life such a half-hearted affair"?[9] Indeed, with mustard gas victims, the very act of nursing was a fraught enterprise. Helen Fairchild, a Red Cross nurse serving with the Pennsylvania Hospital unit at Base Hospital 10 in Le Tréport, wrote home of her first encounter with a rush of gassed patients from nearby Nieuport in July 1917. "Some of the nurses['] eyes were streaming from the vapors," she wrote, "especially in the more closed-in, warm, operating rooms. Doctors and nurses alike have run outside to breathe pure air."[10]

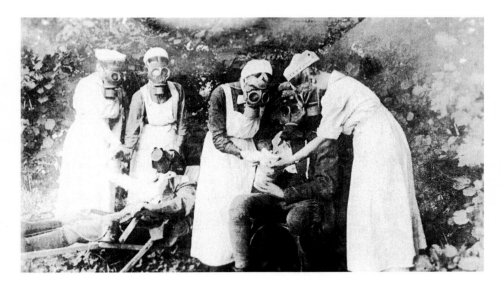

World War I nurses in gas masks treat soldiers after a gas attack.

But exposure to the viscous poison notwithstanding, the nurses did nurse on, pushing themselves to the limit in the effort to provide some measure, *any* measure, of symptom relief. Soldiers in respiratory distress were given oxygen, though many pushed away oxygen masks in the desperate effort to draw in fresh air.[11] Inflamed eyes were repeatedly irrigated with alkaline solution. Respirators, often in short supply,[12] were soaked in hyposulphate and given to patients able to use them. Massive suppurating blisters were drained and the underlying skin cleaned, dried, and treated with antiseptic ointments. At American Base Hospital 10, Fairchild and her fellow nurses washed the "erosive burns" of mustard gas victims with chloride of lime, adding "It's the best we know how to do, but it's not the answer." Then the nurses administered morphine for the pain. But even then, she continued, "there is no end to the screams of the gassed patients when they are touched—even when it is merely their bed sheet touching their skin."[13]

At American Base Hospital 32, on the other hand, where 60 percent of all patients were gas cases,[14] soldiers who had breathed in mustard gas were given a mixture of guiacol, camphor, menthol, alboline, and oils of thyme and eucalyptus that loosened the inflammatory material and caused them to expectorate it. The formula was devised by the Base otolaryngologist, Lafayette Page, but Maude

Essig, an American Red Cross nurse stationed at the hospital, claimed the nurses had a hand in it.[15]

According to Essig, the mixture provided immediate albeit temporary relief to soldiers with burning throats and mouths. But nurses otherwise echoed Helen Fairchild's sense of impotence when it came to making gassed patients comfortable. During the Second Battle of Ypres, when chlorine gas was first used by the Germans, a nurse in a French field hospital in West Flanders recalled the initial wave of gassed troops: "There they lay, fully sensible, choking, suffocating, dying in horrible agonies. We did what we could, but the best treatment for such cases had yet to be discovered, and we felt almost powerless."[16] Shirley Millard was graphic in describing the severe burn patients who rendered nursing futile. "Gas cases are terrible," she wrote at war's end in November 1918.

> They cannot breathe lying down or sitting up. They just struggle for breath, but nothing can be done ... their lungs are gone ... literally burnt out. Some with their eyes and faces entirely eaten away by the gas, and bodies covered with first degree burns. We try to relieve them by pouring oil on them. They cannot be bandaged or even touched.[17]

The nurses may have felt powerless in the face of gassed patients, but "doing what they could" still placed extraordinary demands on them, both physically and emotionally. In October 1917, Newfoundlander Fanny Cluett, a British nursing aide (i.e., a member of Britain's Voluntary Aid Detachment, a VAD) working at 10 General Hospital in Rouen, wrote her mother of "one very sick person, gassed terribly":

> He has oxygen turned on him every hour for 5 minutes; every 4 hrs he has to have gas mixture medicine: then his throat has to be sprayed; he has been awfully miserable this afternoon and evening; the perspiration would pour off him when trying to breathe; I hate to think of him lying there tonight suffering agonies; he has been calling to us every minute to sit with him. He used to say "I am frightened"; every time I passed through the ward, I had to go and sit with him; he could scarcely speak when I came off at 8:30; poor chap! I wonder if he will live until midnight. All his back and one side of his face and a part of his thigh are burnt.[18]

Such were the nursing demands of a single victim of gas warfare whose death was days, if not hours, away. But gassed soldiers never came off the battlefield one at a time. On the contrary, they flooded casualty clearing stations and field hospitals during and after battles in which gas had been deployed. Nurses wrote, variously, of receiving

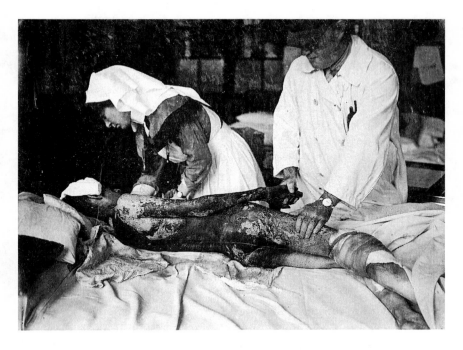

Nursing care of Sergeant Sawyer Spence at Nottingham Hospital, England. Spence, a victim of a mustard gas attack, has severe burns and blisters over most of his body (copyright © John Spence and reprinted with permission).

15 or 18 gassed patients into their wards at a time; of 102 gassed men in a single ward; of "heaps of gassed cases" arriving at a field hospital during the British offensive at Cambrai; of 200 incoming gassed patients overwhelming a field hospital on a given night.[19] Following Germany's release of over 5,700 cylinders of chlorine gas into the Allied lines at Ypres in the spring of 1915, Edith Appleton reported her hospital "filled, emptied and overfilled again. There were men lying on stretchers in the garden, in the grass, and even in the patch known as the duck pond." Those who made it into the hospital, she added, were "very bad indeed and died like poor flies all night."[20] Without letters, diary entries, and postwar reminiscences, it would be difficult to fathom the demands these suffering troops placed on the nurses. Fanny Cluett's "one very sick person, gassed terribly," was hardly alone on her ward. "Nearly all the patients we have got lately on the Medical Lines are gassed," she further informed her mother,

that means their eyes have to be bathed and inhalations of boiling water and Friars balsam; a teaspoonful of balsam to a pint of boiling water. Many of them are burned but not blistered: that is with mustard gas; we do the burns with Baking Soda and Boracic Powders which heal them very quickly.[21]

Whereas soldiers with even the worst of battlefield wounds usually did not complain, wrote Shirley Millard, the severe mustard cases "invariably are beyond endurance and they cannot help crying out." But there were exceptions. Maude Essig wrote of a "star patient," one Leo Moquinn, who "was terribly burned with mustard gas while carrying a pal of his three-quarters of a mile to safety after the gas attack. Except for his back," she added, his "entire body is one third-degree burn. He cannot see and has developed pneumonia and he is delirious." And yet Moquinn never complained, seeking to recover so that he could "finish the 'Boche.'" To Essig's surprise, he recovered well enough to leave the hospital three months after admission and, begging to remain in service in France, rejoined his company before the Armistice was signed. Such was the fate of a chemical burn patient.[22]

Bronchopneumonia, as noted, frequently followed exposure to mustard gas, but Essig's reference to pneumonia alludes to the multitude of infectious diseases that accompanied battlefield wounds and complicated (or prevented) recovery. Absent gas attacks, pneumonia could still be rampant during winter months; gangrene and tetanus were prevalent year-round. Typhoid was partially controlled by the antityphoid serum injections troops received, usually prior to disembarkation but otherwise in the reception huts of clearing stations and field hospitals. But bronchitis, trench fever, diphtheria, cholera, dysentery, meningitis, measles, mumps, erysipelas,[23] and, finally, influenza, simply ran their course. Nurses recorded deaths resulting from various combinations of the foregoing, such as Edith Appleton's "poor little boy, Kerr," who died of gas, pneumonia, and bronchitis.[24] In such instances, there was no point in trying to pinpoint a proximal cause of death.

Infected shrapnel and gunshot wounds could be irrigated or bathed continuously in antiseptics, first developed in the 1870s and packed in sterile dressings available in sealed paper packages since 1893.[25] Widely used antiseptics included carbolic acid, bichloride of mercury, boric acid, and Ensol (chlorinated lime [bleaching powder] and boric acid). "Red lotion" (i.e., mercurochrome) was also at hand; it was first used as a dye in 1889 but Johns Hopkins researchers discovered its antiseptic properties 20 years later.[26] In the preantibiotic era, however, nursing care of systemic infections, including those arising from poison gas, was limited to the same palliatives we employ today: rest, warmth, hydration, nutrition, quinine and phenacetin (no longer in use), all amplified by the nurse's caring, maternal presence.

Trench foot, a combination of fungal infection, frostbite, and poor circulation, was endemic during the winter months, when soldiers lived in trenches flooded with icy water, often waist-high, for days on end. They struggled into clearing stations with feet that were "hideously swollen and purple," feet "that were raw with broken blisters and were wrapped in muddy, dripping bandages."[27] But trench feet, however disabling, at least permitted more active measures. In addition to giving morphine, there was a treatment protocol to follow, such as this one at a British Military Hospital in the winter of 1917:

> We had to rub their feet every morning and every evening with warm olive oil for about a quarter of an hour or so, massage it well in and wrap their feet in cotton wool and oiled silk—all sorts of things just to keep them warm—and then we put big fisherman's socks on them. Their feet were absolutely white, swollen up and dead. Some of their toes dropped off with it, and their feet looked dreadful. We would say, "I'll stick a pin in you. Can you feel it?" Whenever they did feel the pin-prick we knew that life was coming back, and then we'd see a little bit of pink come up and everybody in the ward would cheer.[28]

The dizzying confluence of battlefield injuries, many gangrenous, with the effects of poison gas and intercurrent infectious diseases, threatened to overwhelm the nurses. Reading their diaries and letters, one sees over and over how the nurses' calling, bolstered by the camaraderie of other nurses, surgeons, and orderlies, overpowered resignation and despair. Even in the absence of gas poisoning, multiple injuries on the front were plentiful. In a diary entry of September 14, 1916, Kate Luard referred to the "very special nursing" required by soldiers with multiple severe injuries. She had in mind

> the man with two broken arms has also a wound in the knee—joint in a splint—and has had his left eye removed today. He is nearly crazy. Another man has compound fractures of both legs, one arm, and head, and is quite sensible. Another has both legs amputated, and a compound fracture of [the] arm. These people—as you may imagine—need very special nursing.[29]

Agnes Warner, working out of the hospital at Divonne-Les-Bains on the French-Swiss border, also saw horrid cases of multiple injuries during the summer and fall of 1916. One of her patients, missing his right arm, also "had a bullet in his liver—it is still there—and multiple wounds of head and body." Another was wounded in seven places and one hip was gone.[30] And then, she records her own case of "specializing" (i.e., concentrating on a single patient), in which multiple injuries were compounded by tetanus:

> Today I have been specializing a man who has developed tetanus. I would almost wish that he would die, for he has no hands, and has a great hole in his chest and back, but strange to say he wants to live, is so patient and so full of courage.[31]

Warner's final case is especially revelatory. If one adds to the clusters of battlefield injuries the serious general infections that often accompanied them or resulted from them, one begins to comprehend just what the nurses were up against, and just how special their nursing had to be. When influenza, the deadly Spanish flu, began to swamp clearing stations and hospitals in the spring of 1918, the nurses' initial impulse was simply to add it to the list of challenges to be met with the resources at hand. And they did so, we shall later see, in the knowledge that as many as half of the infected soldiers would die.[32]

I admire the nurses of World War I because they did what was required of them absent any preexisting sense of what they would be required to do, absent, that is, anything approaching a wartime job description. Without internists or infectious disease specialists to fall back on, they subsumed nursing "specialism" within global caregiving identities. This meant they managed multiple war wounds and intercurrent infections, prioritizing among them and continuously adjusting treatment goals in the manner of highly skilled primary care physicians and hospitalists. At the same time, they realized the importance of compassion in the face of their own impotence and despair. Somehow they found time to be present, to slip into a ward with a soldier dying of gas gangrene every few minutes "to do something perfectly useless that might perhaps give a ray of comfort."[33]

It is ironic, given the environment in which they labored and their "patient population" of soldiers in extremis, that nurses embodied the values of primary care medicine, since they assumed the role of primary caregivers obligated to stay with their patients through the course of treatment, to summon senior colleagues and surgeons as needed, and to ease life transitions, whether to recovery, convalescence, lifelong disability, or death.[34] And they did so whatever the weight of multiple assaults on their own bodily and mental integrity.

Nurses, technically noncombatants, suffered alongside the troops. During rushes, their clearing stations, hospitals, and living quarters were under land and air assault and occasionally took direct hits. Nurses contracted infectious diseases, especially diphtheria, dysentery, and flu,[35] during which they often carried on with the aid of simple analgesics until they felt better or worse. In hot weather, such as that encountered by Allied nurses during the Gallipoli campaign of 1915, raging amoebic dysentery overran clearing stations and stationary hospitals, with flies carrying the parasite from infected patients to the nurses, sometimes with fatal results.[36]

When Helen Boylston became feverish in November 1918, a symptom she attributed to diphtheria, she braced herself for a long-awaited evening dance with "quantities of quinine and finally a stiff dose of whiskey, and I felt ready for anything." But not ready enough, it turned out. She collapsed at the dance with a bad chill and had to be carried to her bed. When she went on duty the following day, she became delirious and was lugged off by an orderly and subsequently seen by a doctor. "So here I am," she wrote in her diary. "I've developed a heart and a liver, and am as yellow as a cow-lily. I have to lie flat on my back and be fed. For three days I lay motionless all day long, not caring to move or to speak, I was so tired." Boylston was soon joined by a second nurse with diphtheria, placing the camp "in a panic," with every staff member henceforth given daily throat cultures.[37]

Despite training in the use of gas masks in the event of direct shelling, mask-less nurses suffered the effects of poison gas from daily exposure to patients near whom gas-loaded shells had landed. The volatility of the gas, the manner in which oily fluid clung to and became embedded in clothing, meant that a single gassed soldier could contaminate all the medical personnel—ambulance drivers, orderlies, doctors, and nurses—who came in contact with him. Simply cutting a gassed soldier's clothing off was a fraught enterprise. The nurses' own vulnerability to gas attack and repeated exposure to gassed soldiers lent special intensity to their care of the chemically poisoned. They understood, with Maude Essig and Alice Isaacson, that mustard gas burns meant "terrific suffering," that those gassed and burned by "liquid fire" shells were "very desperately injured, especially about the eyes."[38] Whether infected, wounded, or poisoned, the nurses usually labored on until they collapsed or were so near collapse that medical colleagues ordered them out of the wards and back to their bed or to a "sick sisters" convalescent home for recuperation and a desperately needed time out. The sickest among them were sent to the nearest general hospital. Occasionally they died.[39]

Civil War nurses too eased transitions to death, but their nursing goal during soldiers' final days was to reframe mortal battlefield injury as the promise of a beneficent afterlife. So they stayed with the dying, soliciting final confessions of sinful living, allowing soldiers to reminisce and reflect, and soliciting and writing down words of comfort to sustain family members in believing that their soldier had died a "good death."[40] World War II, on the other hand, witnessed the development of new vaccines, a national blood bank program, the widespread availability of sulfa drugs in 1941 and penicillin in 1944, major advances in the control of shock and bleeding in battlefield surgery, and much greater speed of evacuation of the seriously wounded to European and stateside base hospitals. Taken together, these advances created a buffer between nurses and the prolonged witnessing of soldiers dying in unrelievable pain. And with the buffer came a swagger, a gently sexualized banter with even seriously wounded soldiers, that is worlds removed from the gravely maternal nursing sisters of World War I.

Here, for example is the World War II American army nurse Ruth Haskell, working in an Algerian field hospital during the Allied invasion of North Africa in late 1942. She is talking to a burn victim with one arm "horribly distorted and burned ... fumbling with a match with his one good hand in an effort to light a cigarette."

> "Here, soldier, let me do that," I said as I took the match from his hand.
> "Hello, where did you come from?" he asked. "This isn't such a bad war, after all."
> "Is there anything I can get for you?" I countered. It was a very bad war and we both knew it.
> "You sure can," he said. "A hamburger and a bottle of beer would go right well at this point. How's about it?"
> I looked at him wisely and we both laughed. Was it any wonder one developed a profound respect for boys like these?[41]

And here is June Wandrey, another combat nurse serving in North Africa in 1943, whose stateside duties included care of GIs suffering from pilonidal cysts ("Jeep Seat"). She announced herself to the ward each morning by calling out: "'Bottoms up, fellows.' Thirty plump pairs of smiling buns would turn skyward." And then, after a fellow officer had bared his anatomy for her post-surgical inspection, he ruefully remarked to the accompanying doctor: "'Doc, how can a guy ask a gal out to dinner if she has done his pelvic dressings?' The Major smiled, winked at me, and said, 'Do you want to make a bet?'"[42] The American nurses of World War I record no such easy banter; it was not of their time and place. More characteristic is the incident related by Indianan Maude Essig in a diary entry of November 5, 1918, a mere six days before the Armistice was signed. Three officers grateful for their nursing care in Essig's Base Hospital 32 took her and two other nurses out for a farewell dinner before returning to the Front. But the nurses did not appreciate their drinking to excess and insisted on leaving them in mid-celebration. "I guess they thought us a queer lot," Essig wrote, "but I hope they will remember us as decent women."[43]

None of this—not the banter, the innuendos, the asides—is to minimize the physical and emotional burdens of World War II nurses, indeed, of nurses working under battlefield conditions in any war. One has only to read accounts of army nurses who served in the South Pacific during 1944 and 1945, working in unbearable tropical heat in primitive open-sided tent hospitals, learning to run IV lines and administer intravenous anesthesia on the spot, to appreciate their courage and dedication to duty. When supply ships ran aground on coral reefs, nurses on the island of Lemnos struggled to keep patients alive with next to no equipment or medicine. One such nurse, Ellen Dellane, based in Saipan, recalls having only a single thermometer to share among a group of diphtheria patients.[44] The primitive nursing conditions in the Philippines, especially before the delayed arrival of supply ships, evokes the conditions encountered by Canadian and Australian nurses on islands off the Gallipoli peninsula in 1916 and on the swampy, mosquito-infested Greek island of Salonika in the same year.

But there are fundamental differences. The American nurses of World War II were of a different generation; they entered military nursing beneficiaries of the socially liberating 1920s; they joined an Army Nursing Corps that was far larger, better organized, and more militarily influential than that of their predecessors. Their GI patients were "boys" in the familiar sense of brothers, former classmates, boyfriends and lovers. Bearing up under the weight of serious injuries, massive burns among them, the GIs were, as Haskell remarked, "swell kids," one and all.[45] The nurses of World War I also claimed patients as their "boys," but usually absent the companionable gendered gloss. A nurse's boys, regardless of age differences, were usually surrogate sons because, after all, they were someone else's sons back home.[46]

In World War II, chemical weapons were used regularly in U.S. Army Air Corps strategic bombing campaigns in both European and Pacific theaters. But they were not deployed against infantry on the battlefield. In World War I, on the other hand, ground troops injured during gas attacks were often in agony, blinded, struggling to breathe, literally coughing up tracheal and bronchial tissue. For the beleaguered nurses, these patients were not soldier boys whose spirits could be lifted by deftly feminized attention; rather, they were boy soldiers, children whose only desire was for mothering that would ease the pain, if only through morphinized sleep that permitted a peaceful death.

The nurses of World War I who "nursed" severely gassed soldiers suffered themselves, and their suffering was unmediated and visceral. They could not sustain themselves and their patients with the naturalistic view of the afterlife popular during the Civil War.[47] Nor did they have the benefit of World War II technology and organization to shield them, at least partially, from the experiential onslaught of mortally wounded soldiers suffering as they died. For the nurses of the Great War, it was less death per se than the agony of dying—from infected battle wounds compounded by systemic infections, gas gangrene, poison gas, rushed amputations followed by reinfection and blood loss—that took them to the existential no-man's-land we encountered in the writings of Mary Borden and Ellen La Motte.[48]

And it was the dying of sons, their own surrogate sons, that made the agony of dying boys their own. More than their sisters in the world war to follow, the nurses of World War I embraced Florence Nightingale's vision of nursing as woman's work, which for Nightingale meant that any woman could be a nurse. The gendered belief that nursing summoned skills that were intrinsic to women's domestic sphere, especially mothering, carried over to the next generation of nurse educators. In her influential textbooks on nursing practice of the 1890s, for example, Isabel Hampton Robb, the first superintendent of the Johns Hopkins Hospital Training School, retained Nightingale's belief that nursing care, however enlarged by the growth of scientific medicine, remained woman's work. She reminded nursing students, for example, that hospital etiquette obliged them to treat the ward as a home, with the head nurse the head of the family. "As at home we should never dream of receiving a visitor seated," she admonished, "so a nurse should not remain seated when any one enters her ward." And further, for all their training, nurses, for Robb, continued to transform their work environments in distinctly feminine ways. The communities and institutions where nurses toiled, that is, would always "show forth the influence of that sweet ordering, and arrangement and decision that are woman's chief prerogatives."[49] This is the imagery of Civil War nursing, when experienced nurses complained that the return of convalescent soldiers to their regiments broke up their "little households"; they returned from leave "homesick" to get back to their work.[50]

Borden, La Motte, Vera Brittain, and countless confrères bore witness to the enormous disparity between modern industrialized slaughter and the meager resources of a military medical establishment that began the war looking back to the last century rather than forward to the new one. This disparity guaranteed that the nurses would often be impotent as womanly caregivers in the face of gangrenous wounds, suppurating stumps, multiple infections, and especially the effects of poison gas. The obligation to bear witness to a protracted and anguished dying that could not be nursed into womanly submission—this was the nurses' own no man's land. Their feeling of impotence, which became more profound still with the arrival of deadly influenza in the final months of the war, was conducive neither to the resigned quietude of the Civil War nurses who preceded them nor the confident, sometimes playful brio of the professionalized World War II nurses who followed them. In the Great War, the womanly component of nursing care was that of mothers for sons, and many nurses lived with a sense of maternal failure in the face of suffering that could not be eased and lives that could not be saved in a war that could not be maternally transformed.

The letters and diaries of World War I nurses who wrote about their nursing work are suffused with maternalism, including acceptance of the more than honorific designation "mother" the wounded bestowed on them. This maternalism is front and center in the letters of Kate Norman Derr, a French-trained American Red Cross nurse who served with the rank of Lieutenant in a French Field Hospital near the trenches of the Marne. For Derr, patients were all her children, and she became their *petite mère*, their little mother.[51] But the same need for mothering appears in the letters and diaries of many others. In this respect, the nurses of the Great War looked back to their forebears in the Civil War, the untrained hospital volunteers who came to their nursing role as mothers intent on providing the kindness and caring that hardened military surgeons could not. There is little difference between Louisa May Alcott, for whom the patients were "my big babies" and Kate Norman Derr, who, come Christmas time, 1915, refused a holiday leave because "mothers who love their children don't go off and leave them with empty stockings then."[52]

But there is an important difference: In World War I maternal nursing care was not simply a matter of Civil War–era kindness and solicitousness, of struggles with corrupt quartermasters to keep the wounded warm and decently fed. Rather, their maternal care opened to a mode of perception that provided privileged access to industrialized warfare in all its monstrous destructiveness. The battlefield nurses of World War I, some of whom were deeply religious, could not rest content with the maternalism of their Civil War forebears. Consider Hannah Ropes, for example, for whom her charge was "to do my Master's work; the poor privates are my special children for the present; I never wash their hard, worn, and sore feet without a sweet memory of Him who gave us the example."[53] Nor could they summon the stridency of Mary Ann Bickerdyke ("Mother Bickerdyke"), who famously answered a surgeon inquiring on the source of her authority during the Battle of Shiloh with, "On the authority of Lord God Almighty, have you anything that outranks that?"[54] Rather, the nurses of the Great War were horrified at what their maternal gaze let them see. The Scottish novelist and Red Cross nurse Sarah Macnaughtan, who nursed the wounded in Belgium, France, and Russia in 1914 and 1915, gave voice to this gendered futility in a diary entry written before her death in 1916:

> The loss of the lives of their sons will always appear to women to be too high a price to pay for anything the world contains or is able to produce. The whole idea of the value of life is inherent in them…. In the almost unbearable pain of loss she demands to know, what is the logical connection between boys with their lungs shot through and their heads blown off, and a madman's

greed for territory and power? Sitting by some sick-bed when the candles are burning low, she seeks some explanation of the sheer, horrible idiocy of the whole thing.[55]

For many nurses of the Great War, it was the severely gassed who brought home the idiocy of the whole thing with a terrifying immediacy. But their life-altering experience of the gassed was not shared by others. After the Armistice the action of poison gas and the agony of its victims were muted by the medical press. In 1925, for example, the editors of the *British Medical and Surgical Journal*, in an editorial on "Gas in Warfare," voiced agreement with the noted biologist J. B. S. Haldane, who had written that the use of gas and other chemical agents in warfare "were both more humane and more efficient than the older weapons." "The time may come," the editor opined, "when rifles, machine guns and explosives will be considered barbarous and inhumane as compared with gas." And in 1940, when the next world war was already upon Europe, Leon Goldman and Glenn Cullen, writing in the *Journal of the American Medical Association*, announced that

> the truth of the matter is that there are relatively few residuals from chemical warfare and certainly not those horrible ones following shrapnel, gunshot wounds and the like. If any kind of warfare could be called "humane," chemical warfare warrants such a term.[56]

If "gas discipline" were improved, they added, poison gas casualties in the next war would be greatly reduced. But then, even back in August 1918, the *British Medical Journal* believed the sequelae to gas poisoning had been "greatly exaggerated." The "persistent and troublesome vomiting" of gas victims, it editorialized, was "undoubtedly neurotic." Further, prolonged stays in hospitals should be avoided, he added, since such stays were "particularly apt to exaggerate the neurotic conditions, which are then difficult to overcome.... Means should be taken to convince the patient that the condition is not serious."[57] Seven years later, in the editorial on "Gas in Warfare," the *BMJ*'s verdict was that "neurasthenic [neurotic] conditions" were "responsible for a considerable part of the disability alleged to result from gassing." Readers were forewarned that "few of the cases that receive a pension will ever admit a subsequent improvement or cure." The key was to prevent the large percentage of gas victims whose symptoms were "functional" (i.e., neurotic) from claiming disability in the first place. This, according to John A. Ryle, echoing the position of the *BMJ*, was simply a matter of "reeducation and persuasion." Gas poisoning, it turned out, was not so bad after all.[58]

The battlefield nurses of the war knew better. They had triaged and treated the soldiers who struggled back to field hospitals after exposure to mustard gas; they arrived with corroded respiratory systems and seared lungs, gasping for air, blinded, with eyes on fire with conjunctivitis and photophobia. The vomiting that developed four to eight hours later was far from "neurotic"; it was part of a symptom complex, and could be "persistent and intractable."[59] Septic bronchopneumonia, as noted above, was another part of the complex, and usually set in within two days.

In the summer of 1917, the nurses at No. 12 General Hospital on the outskirts of Rouen struggled with a gas victim whose paroxysms of coughing came every minute and a half "by the clock," and who had not slept in four days. To quiet him, they rigged up a croup tent under which they took turns holding a small stove that heated a croup kettle from which the soldier could breathe the steam. When sleep finally came, they were "ready to get down on their knees in gratitude, his anguish had been so terrible to watch." To their head nurse, Julia Stimson, they remarked that "they could not wish the Germans any greater unhappiness than to have them have to witness the sufferings of a man like that and know that they had been the cause of it."[60] The British nursing aide and budding littérateur Vera Brittain, struggling along at British General Hospital No. 24 at Étaples, expressed the same sentiment but aimed it at those on the home front who glorified the war and urged its continuation:

> I wish those people who write so glibly about this being a holy War, and the orators who talk so much about going on no matter how long the War lasts and what it may mean, could see a case—to say nothing of 10 cases—of mustard gas in its early stages—could see the poor things burnt and blistered all over with great mustard-colored suppurating blisters, with blind eyes—sometimes temporally [*sic*], sometimes permanently—all sticky and stuck together, and always fighting for breath, with voices a mere whisper, saying that their throats are closing and they know they will choke. The only thing one can say is that such severe cases don't last long; either they die soon or else improve—usually the former; they certainly never reach England in the state we have them here, and yet people persist in saying that God made the War, when there are such inventions of the Devil about.[61]

For the nurses of World War I, bearing witness to the unrelievable agony of severe gassing was, along with the untreatable suffering of those struck down by influenza in the fall of 1918, the worst assault they bore. "It is dreadful to be impotent, to stand by grievously stricken men it is impossible to help, to see the death-sweat gathering on young faces, to have no means of easing their last moments. This is the nearest to Hell I have yet been." This is the voice of an anonymous British Red Cross nurse, unsettled by the dying Belgian soldiers she encountered on ambulance runs in the fields of West Flanders in the winter of 1915. The American nurses at No. 12 General Hospital brushed up against the same hell, and they could think of no better retribution than making enemy combatants bear witness to what they had witnessed. During its first week of operation in the summer of 1917, American Base Hospital No. 10, an untested unit from the University of Pennsylvania based in Le Tréport, received 1,400 casualties during its first week of operation, most of whom were either surgical or mustard gas cases. The gas patients, recalled head nurse Margaret Dunlap, were "horrible pictures of misery" and provided the unit with its "first soul-harassing introduction to the indescribable barbarity by which war is inflicted upon the individual soldier."[62]

But souls can be harassed without succumbing to torment. The nurses of World War I were not stymied by impotence in the face of suffering that arose from the indescribable barbarity they beheld and then, despite themselves, tried to describe. On the contrary, they remained soulful amid the agony of gassed patients, many of whom, they knew full well, could not be comforted much less saved. They labored on to the breaking point in the service of soldiers who all too often were already broken. This makes them warriors of care and, in a devotion to patients that was literally and not metaphorically selfless, heroes of the first rank.

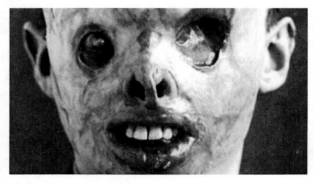

Mustard gas facial burns, ne plus ultra of the "indescribable barbarity" of the Great War.

5

Shell Shock

"They were very pathetic, these shell-shocked boys."[1]

Every war has mental casualties, but each war has its own way of understanding and treating them. Each war, that is, has its own nomenclature for what it understands as combat-related mental disorder, all of which we now gather under the rubric of psychiatric diagnosis.[2] As far back as the seventeenth century, Swiss physicians wrote of the deep despair—now we call it depression—of conscripted Swiss troops forced to serve in France; the young men appeared to be dying, sometimes literally, of homesickness fueled by strange foreign customs and the absence of maternal care. During the Napoleonic era, nostalgia was rife among young French recruits transposed from the small villages of western France to the privations and enforced idleness of military camps. Actual epidemics of nostalgia broke out in both the Army of the Rhine in 1793 and the Army of the Alps in 1799.[3] By 1800, the British navy recognized the disabling hopelessness described in Swiss, Spanish, and French accounts as a condition to which sailors on campaigns were especially vulnerable; the sailors, according to their surgeons, had succumbed to "melancholia."

During the American Civil War, nostalgia was widely diagnosed, but a new term, "irritable heart" (aka "soldier's heart" or "Da Costa's Syndrome" or "effort syndrome") was coined just after the war to describe a different kind of syndrome. Soldiers with the condition experienced uncontrollable shivering and trembling accompanied by rapid heartbeat and difficulty breathing. In the 10-week Spanish-American War of 1898, American soldiers who broke down mentally amid heat, bugs, bullets, and rampant typhoid fever were diagnosed with "tropical weakness." The following year, Boer War physicians recurred to irritable heart—both the term and the symptom cluster—which became a major cause of invalidism among British troops. Interestingly, the highest incidence of irritable heart in South Africa was among orderlies in the Royal Army Medical Corps—a result, it was surmised, of the great distances medical field units had to traverse to provide support to widely dispersed troop actions. Nor did the heavy medical gear carried by the orderlies during the long treks help matters, heart-wise.[4]

And this brings us to World War I, the war that bequeathed the venerable diagnosis of shell shock, a term that outlasted the war and, beginning with the Great Depression of 1929, passed into America's cultural vocabulary as a signifier of overwhelming, indeed paralyzing, distress.[5] In the Great War, however, shell shock was a mental disability, and the sheer number of those so diagnosed dwarfed the mental casualties of preceding wars and posed a genuine threat to manpower requirements of the combatants. Britain in particular was hard hit. By December 1914, 7–10 percent of British officers and 3–4 percent of British troops, all uninjured, were "nervous and mental shock" casualties. At the Battle of the Somme in the summer of 1916 as many as 40 percent of all British casualties were psychiatric, i.e., evacuated to Britain as shell shocked in the global sense.[6]

At first the nurses of World War I were no less baffled by the variable expressions of shell shock—most instances of which, it was soon learned, arose some distance from exploding shells at the front—than the doctors. The term was coined in early 1915 by the British physician and psychologist Charles Myers, then part of a volunteer medical unit in France. Myers quickly realized the term was a misnomer: He coined it after seeing three soldiers whose similar psychological symptoms followed the concussive impact of artillery shells bursting at close range. In these cases, he surmised, the high-frequency vibrations caused by exploding shells might cause "an invisibly fine 'molecular' commotion in the brain," and the commotion, in turn, led to symptoms of dissociation.[7] But he soon discovered that many men with the same symptoms were nowhere near exploding shells.

By the time he was appointed "Consultant Specialist in Nervous Shock" to the British Army in March 1915, Myers believed shell shock symptoms were entirely mental in nature. The French Army was less generous. It considered traumatized soldiers malingerers and kept them near the front to dissuade others from following suit. The German Army, for its part, viewed soldiers who broke down and developed symptoms as unworthy and unpatriotic; they burdened them with a diagnosis otherwise reserved for women: hysteria. German officers had it better. They were given the far less pejorative label "neurasthenic," a diagnostically polite way of saying they had succumbed to nervous exhaustion; in a word, their nerves were shot.

In May 1917, the American psychiatrist Thomas Salmon, with the approval of the War Department, traveled to England to observe how the British treated their shell-shocked soldiers. He returned home convinced that what the British termed shell shock and considered a category of war neurosis, was a real disorder, not to be taken for malingering. As such, it was a disorder amenable to psychological treatment, especially if it were promptly administered. Like others, he questioned the term "shell shock," given the well-established fact that only a small number of cases occurred in the presence of shell fire.

But the problem of war neurosis was a real and pressing concern, especially because soldiers so incapacitated had very favorable prognoses for returning to combat duty within a period of weeks or months. The key, as Salmon saw it, was to cordon off all the neuropsychiatric cases from the general medical population in special hospitals. "Few more hopeful cases exist in the medical services," he reported, "than those suffering from the war neuroses grouped under the term 'shell shock' when treated in special hospitals by physicians and nurses familiar with the nature of functional nervous diseases and with their management." Further, since successful treatment of shell shock cases required treatment as soon as possible to avoid giving affected soldiers the "coloring of invalidism," Salmon recommend that select base hospitals establish neuro-psychiatric wards in forward areas nearer the front.[8]

Salmon was the Medical Director of the National Committee for Mental Hygiene, so his report to the Surgeon General carried weight. Without delay, the U.S. Army began making arrangements for treating the mental casualties that, Salmon predicted, could flood overseas and stateside hospitals following America's entry into the war.[9]

Nurses already at the front and the American contingent shortly to arrive were unconcerned with the animated debate among physicians on the nature of shell shock. Was it, according to Myers' original formulation, a kind of brain concussion that resulted from the blast force of exploding shells? A neurological response to prolonged fear? A psychological reaction to the impact of industrial warfare? A product of nervous shock analogous to that suffered by victims of railway accidents in the later nineteenth century?[10] Or perhaps it was a Freudian-type "war neurosis" in which trauma at the front plugged into traumas the soldier had suffered earlier in life. The nurses did not care. Theirs was the everyday world of distressed soldiers, whose symptoms, often florid, overlay profound anxiety, and whose reliving of trauma and its aftermath occurred throughout the day and night. Theirs, that is, was the world of containment and short-term management.

In undertaking the management part, the nurses could be bemused, good-naturedly patronizing, at times irritated. Shell shock

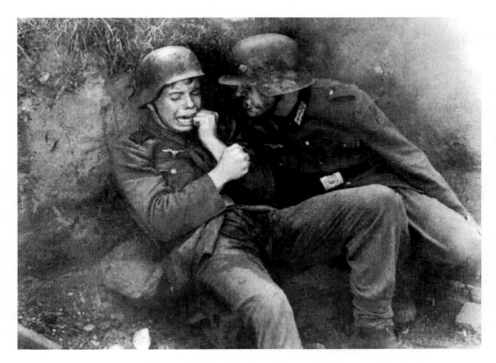

A young German soldier who has broken down in his trench being comforted by a comrade.

victims, after all, made unusual demands on nurses and their aides. The patients, it seemed, were always falling out of bed and otherwise "shaking and stammering and looking depressed and scared." Simple tasks like serving meals could be a project, as attested to by the British volunteer nurse (i.e., VAD) Grace Bagnold, who, prior to becoming a nursing aide in 1915, worked as an orderly at a London convalescent home. There, she recalled,

> one of the things I was told was that when I was serving meals ... always to put the plate down very carefully in front of them and to let them see me do it. If you so much as put a plate down in front of them in the ordinary way, when they weren't looking, the noise made them almost jump through the roof—just the noise of a plate being put on a table with a cloth on it?[11]

Accommodation by the orderlies at meal time paled alongside the constant burden on ward nurses who had to calm hospitalized shell shock soldiers when exploding shells and overhead bombs rocked the hospital, taking patients back to the front and scenes of battlefield trauma, with the anxiety attendant to what they had seen or done, or had done to them or to others. And both, perhaps, paled alongside the burden of nurses in the ambulance trains that transported the shell shocked out of the trenches or off the battlefield. "It was a horrible thing," wrote the ambulance nurse Clair Elise Tisdall,

> because they sometimes used to get these attacks, rather like epileptic fits in a way. They became quite unconscious, with violent shivering and shaking, and you had to keep them from banging themselves about too much until they came round again. The great thing was to keep them from falling off the stretchers, and for that reason we used to take just one at a time in the ambulance ... these were the so-called milder cases; we didn't carry the dangerous ones. They always tried to keep that away from us and they came in a separate part of the train.[12]

The dangerous cases were the "hopeless mental cases" destined, Tisdall recalled, for "a special place," i.e., a mental hospital, in England termed a "neurasthenic centre." But how to tell the difference? The line between mild and severe cases of shell shock was subjectively drawn and constantly fluctuating. Soldiers who arrived in the hospital with some combination of headaches, tremors, a stutter, memory loss, and vivid flashback dreams might become psychosomatically blind, deaf, or mute. Or they might develop paralyzed or spastic limbs after settling into base hospitals and the care of nurses.

In their diaries and letters home, nurses' characterizations of the shell shocked are often patronizing and can sound unkind. For Julia Stimson, they were one of "the most pitiful groups." "The other night," she wrote home in June 1917, "the explosion of shells could be distinctly heard, and almost all these cases shook as though they were having convulsions all night." Amy Trent, an AEF nurse serving with Base Hospital No. 3 in Montpon-Ménestérol in southwestern France, was no less judgmental a year later. In a letter posted to the editor of the *American Journal of Nursing* and published in the issue of September 1918, she informed stateside colleagues that the shell shock cases, "require patience. It is pathetic to see how nervous and generally unstrung they are." In her diary Dorothea Crewdson referred to them as "dithery shell shocks" and "old doddering shell shocks." A patient who without warning got out of bed and raced down the hall clad only in his nightshirt was a "dotty poor dear." "It is sad to see them," wrote Edith Appleton. "They dither like palsied old men, and talk all the time about their mates who were blown to bits, or their mates who were wounded and never brought in. The whole scene is burnt into their brains and they can't get rid of the sight of it."[13]

Dorothea Crewdson too, for all her brio, understood only too well why the shell shocked were dotty and dithering. It was all about fear and shattered nerves. What appeared on the surface as comical dottiness was a desperate search for cover. Nighttime bombing raids and the alarms that signaled them were the worst:

> All the poor shell shocks will be dancing about with fright if an enemy does begin his money tricks. They were much upset by the last raid and lots of them are as bad as ever again. Most pathetic, poor things. Their nerves seem to have absolutely gone to pieces.[14]
>
> Poor shell shocks went scuttling off, like a lot of rabbits, from the marquees to the building. These night raids put the wind up and their shattered nerves won't stand the shock at all.[15]

◆　◆　◆

Yet, looked at more closely, even such patronizing descriptions have an air of reassuring normalcy about them. Viewed historically, there is difficulty not only distinguishing mild and severe cases of shell shock but identifying cases of shell shock per se. Perhaps one reason the nurses could not be bothered with debates about the etiology of shell shock was that they saw early on exactly how hazy the diagnosis was. It was hazy even to the neurologists and psychiatrists who theorized about it. But for the nurses there was another consideration, a fact of nursing life we have addressed in other contexts: the multiple serious injuries that brought the wounded to casualty clearing stations and field hospitals off the front. Shell-shocked soldiers, that is, were often wounded in other ways, and it remained obscure (and, in the here and now of CCSs and field hospitals, clinically irrelevant) whether a condition called "shell shock" coexisted with traumatizing battlefield injuries or simply gave urgent, hopefully transient, expression to them. Which soldiers were actually shell shocked and which simply in the throes of an injury-induced breakdown or a breakdown pure and simple?

The Canadian nurse Sophie Hoerner, stationed at No. 1 Canadian General Hospital in early 1915, wrote home repeatedly of the "dreadful suffering" caused by bursting shrapnel, which "rips, tears, lacerates and penetrates the tissue in a horrible manner." "Some of them go right to pieces," she continued. "Their nerve has gone and they cry like babies. Others just stare and say nothing, have such a vacant look."[16] The American Red Cross (ARC) nurse Shirley Millard, the Oregonian who served in a French military hospital after America's entry into the war, recollected "an English boy in the fracture ward" who simply "went insane. He tried to choke one of the English nurses. She struggled with him and the orderlies rushed over and pinned him down. Poor kid! They had to put him in a strait-jacket. I wonder what will happen to him."[17]

Are soldiers who awaken to devastating wounds shell shocked in any meaningful psychological sense? It is impossible to believe that all who experienced regressions or violent outbursts or defensive withdrawal in the immediate aftermath of such injuries were shell shocked or insane in any credible diagnostic sense. The sheer severity of the injuries and attendant pain mitigate the need to excavate underlying mental conflicts or point the finger at the wounded soldier's "psychopathic predisposition" or "psychopathic reaction" or "fixed ideas" in the manner of wartime Freudians.[18]

A different kind of example comes from another Canadian nurse, Kate Wilson, a farm girl from rural Ontario whose military odyssey took her to hospitals in England, France, and the Greek island of Lemnos. She writes here from British Casualty Clearing Station No. 44 at Puchevillers, near the Somme, in early July 1916. On arrival, she landed in a "ward of horrors," where she was responsible for 48 wounded, of whom "possibly ten might live to see the base hospital." And then she describes what for her were the most harrowing cases—the head cases:

> A boy would come in with all his senses, and suddenly I would hear a scream, and would find that he had gone absolutely insane, often with all his bandages torn off, and his wound hemorrhaging, with particles of his brain oozing out of the open wound. Immediately he would be moved to an empty tent.[19]

The example is extreme; it is doubtful nurses at the time would have equated the hysterical outburst of this traumatically injured, probably dying soldier with a case of shell shock. But there were other examples where the diagnostic ordering is less clear. Wilson also mentions a case of shell shock accompanied by a hemorrhaging amputated limb and another admitted with "erratic heart action."[20] Was the latter a case of shell shock or a transient panic reaction to frightening cardiac symptoms? Or perhaps he was a case of "soldier's heart" (DaCosta's syndrome) with the symptoms associated with *that* hazy diagnosis. And were Wilson's patients on the same spectrum as the otherwise uninjured patient who simply "shakes all the time"?[21] Or those soldiers, also deemed shell shocked, who were violent on arrival at the CCS because they believed they were still on the battlefield?[22] Edith Appleton, we have seen, considered soldiers shell shocked who talked continuously with their mates about the horror they had experienced on the front. Here she elaborates further on these cases:

> The whole scene is burnt into their brains and they can't get rid of the sight of it. One rumpled, raisin-faced old fellow said his job was to take bombs up to the bombers, and sometimes going through the trenches he had to push past men with their arms blown off or horribly wounded, and they would yell at him, "Don't touch me," but he had to get past, because the fellows must have their bombs. Then he would stand on something wobbly and nearly fall down—and see it was a dying or dead man, half covered in mud.[23]

There is no question that Appleton's soldiers have been traumatized; today, we see them suffering from PTSD. But are they shell shocked in the sense of Charles Myers, Gordon Holmes, and Lewis Yealland? Muteness, bear in mind, was a major symptom of shell shock. For Appleton's soldiers, the very ability to perseverate among themselves about what they experienced suggests an effort at working through trauma in the therapeutic milieu of a hospital ward of fellow sufferers. Are they psychiatric cases? Undoubtedly. Are they shell shocked? Only in the loosest descriptive sense. One can be traumatized without being "shocked" in either the neurological or psychodynamic senses of the term current throughout the Great War.

For the British VAD Vera Brittain, the signs of shell shock had nothing to do with perseveration or shaking. Rather they were withdrawal, manifested in mood, body language, skin tone, and "deathly cold." Following a German bombing raid, her brother Edward was diagnosed with shell shock and hospitalized at Fishmongers' Hall, a military hospital for officers in London. Vera visited him in February 1916 and offered this characterization:

> On my next afternoon off duty I went to Fishmongers' Hall, and found him [Edward], in a green dressing-gown, huddled over a gas-fire with a rug across his knees. Though the little wound on his left cheek was almost healed, he still shuddered from the deathly cold that comes after shell-shock; his face was grey with a queer, unearthly pallor, from which his haunted eyes glowed like twin points of blue flame in their sunken sockets.[24]

In more severe cases, the withdrawal became vacancy, to which a tic could be added. The example is from the British ambulance driver Helen Zenna Smith's autobiographical novel of 1930, *Not So Quiet....Stepdaughters of War.* Wounded soldiers able to sit up in her ambulance, she recounts, could tell her many a thing during the long rides back to the hospital. But not the shell shocked:

> No, not shell-shock. The shell-shock cases take it more quietly as a rule, unless they are suddenly startled. Let me find you an example. Ah, the man they are bringing out now. The one staring straight ahead at nothing ... twitching, twitching, twitching, each limb working in a different direction, like a Jumping Jack worked by a jerking string.[25]

New Englander Helen Dore Boylston, a graduate of the nursing program at Massachusetts General Hospital and member of the Harvard Medical Unit, conflated shell shock with a situationally induced panic attack. Working at a British hospital, she recorded an incident from July 1916 when German planes bombed her hut several times, leaving many of her patients badly wounded. Her medical officer was with her, but rather than helping with the wounded, he crawled under a bed in the corner and had what she termed a "shell shock fit."[26]

For the nurses, then, shell shock was a heuristic; it meant whatever it was called on to mean in particular circumstances. They made a general distinction between shell shock and madness, even though displays of mad behavior were often imputed to the shell shocked. In the CCSs and field hospitals, the pragmatics of management and containment trumped etiologic considerations. No doubt they would have scoffed at some of the more arcane theorizing that physicians and psychiatrists resorted to. What could they do, for example, with Freud's claim that with shell-shocked soldiers, "the danger of external violence might manifest itself as the ego's fear of an internal enemy"? Or with his student Karl Abraham's conjecture that the shell shocked were incipiently neurotic, with restricted sexual activity that derived from "libido inhibited by fixations"?[27] Such pearls of psychoanalytic theorizing—Freud had never treated a case of shell shock, and Abraham's very limited exposure came as a general surgeon—were worthless to battlefield nurses. They simply nursed on, relying on intuitive understanding, commonsense psychology, and compassion. And, all things considered, they did amazingly well. Arguably, they were among the first modern health care professionals to assume the working identity of supportive psychotherapists. This was especially true of nurses whose backgrounds in social work and social services led to assignment to military hospitals devoted to shell shock patients. Some, such as Edith Ambrose, a member of the first graduating class of New York's Presbyterian Hospital who then received public health training at Teachers College, expressly requested such assignment. In April 1918, she wrote Clara Noyes, then head of the ARC's department of nursing, that she was "perhaps as well equipped to do psychiatric work as any nurse, if not better," citing five years' experience doing "re-educational work for all kinds of functional nervous disorders."[28]

• • •

It is in the containment aspects of their work that the nurses evinced the same caring acceptance of shell-shocked patients that they brought to all their patients. After all, shell-shocked patients, however they presented, were wounded soldiers, and their suffering was as real and intense as that of comrades with bodily wounds. The nursing historian Christine Hallett, who writes of the World War I nurses with great insight and sympathy, credits nurses working with the shell shocked with an almost preternatural psychoanalytic sensibility in containing the trauma that underlay their symptoms. The nurses, she claims, aligned themselves with the patients, however disruptive their outbursts and enactments, since they "sensed that insanity would be a 'normal' response for any man who fully realized the deliberateness of the destruction that had been unleashed on him." Hence, she continues,

> nurses conspired with their patients to "ignore" or "forget" the reality of warfare until it was safe to remember. In this way they ameliorated the effect of the "psychic splintering" caused by trauma. They contained the effects of this defensive fragmentation—the "forgetting" and the "denial"—until patients were able to confront their memories, incorporate them as part of themselves and become "whole" beings again.[29]

It is easy to follow Hallett in her insistence that nurses usually ignored the directive not to "spoil" shell-shocked patients. All too often, they let themselves get involved with them at the expense of maintaining professional distance and control of their wards.[30] But then the nurses were equally caring and equally prone to personal connection with all their patients, mental or not. They were not psychotherapists, and the dizzying demands of their long days and nights did not permit empathic engagement in any psychoanalytic sense, beyond the all-too-human realization that the shell shocked had experienced something so horrible as to require a gentleness, a lightness of touch, and a willingness to accept strange adaptive defenses that, with the right kind of nursing, would probably peel away slowly over time. This approach, interestingly, parallels the dramatic fall in shell shock rates that grew out of the third battle of Ypres (Passchendaele) when, following the lead of the British neurologist Gordon Holmes, the Allied armies adopted an approach to shell shock that respected the individual's coping skills, and allowed these skills, over time, to dissipate the shock reaction.[31] Just such an approach was the nurses' forte. Here, for example, is one of Hallett's examples of "emotional containment" on the part of the Australian army nurse Elsie Steadman:

> It was very interesting work, some of course could not move, others could not speak, some had lost their memory, and did not even know their own names, others again had very bad jerks and twitching. Very careful handling these poor lads needed, for supposing a man was just finding his voice, to be spoken to in any way that was not gentle and quiet the man "was done," and you would have to start all over again to teach him to talk, the same things applied to walking, they must be allowed to take their time.[32]

This sensitivity, this "very careful handling" of the shell shocked, was no different than the sensitivity of the mealtime orderlies, who knew to "put the plate down very carefully in front of them," always making sure that the shell shocked saw them do it. And of course there were accommodations out of the ordinary, a remarkable example of which comes from Julia Stimson, the American chief nurse of British Base Hospital 21. Stimson, an amateur violinist, related "an interesting little incident" to her parents in late November 1917. It began when a patient knocked on her door and asked for the matron:

> He was so wobbly he almost had to lean up against the wall. "Somebody told me," he said, "that you had a violin. I am a professional violinist and I have not touched a violin for five months, and today I couldn't stand it any longer, so I got up out of bed to come and find you." I made him come in and sit down. As it happened I had a new violin and bow, which had been bound for our embryo orchestra, here in my office. The violin was not tuned up, but that didn't matter. The man had it in shape in no time and then he began to play and how he could play! We let him take the violin down to his tent, and later sent him some of my music. He was a shell shock, and all the evening and the next few days until he was sent to England he played to rapt audiences of fellow patients.[33]

Another inventive shell shock remedy comes from Kate Wilson, who recounts an incident in Boulogne at Canadian General Hospital No. 3 in the spring of 1916:

> Sister Pat accidentally stumbled on a cure for at least one shell shocked victim in her ward who had lost his power of speech. One morning coming on duty, looking as usual, like a pink rose, she hurried to her service table, threw back the lid of a small tin box that she used to hold her pencils and small articles, and out jumped a small mouse! Pat gave an unearthly scream, and the shell-shock case followed suit. Sitting straight up in his cot, with the perspiration running down his face and shaking in every limb he cried "Sister, I can talk!" And with that reaction he burst into tears. Little did the wag who had caught the mouse and placed it in the box realize the good deed that he had done that day.[34]

What have we here if not a benignly attenuated version of the *torpillage* (torpedoing) of Clovis Vincent in France and the "faradization" of Edgar Adrian and Lewis Yealland in London—primitive and sometimes brutal applications of electric shock to the paralyzed or dysfunctional body part of a shell-shocked soldier. The theory underlying this approach was that powerful countershock could overcome the symptoms of shock. According to the psychiatrists and neurologists who espoused this approach, the symptoms of shell shock—muteness, blind-ness, paralysis—were simply products of the soldier's fear-driven "auto-suggestion." It followed that cure could be effected through an even stronger countersuggestion provided by the physician. The method to this end was disarmingly simple: Doctors simply told patients, with the full weight of medical authority, that they *would* get better and then that they *had* gotten better. Their medical judgment was then driven home by the electrodes, presented to patients as a veritable magic wand that most assuredly would effect the cure. If a patient's paralyzed limb was shocked with an electrode, for example, the patient would experi-ence sensation and "move" that limb. The doctor would seize on the movement to persuade the patient that he was well on the road to cure, indeed, that he was cured already. The same was true of mute patients, for whom faradization of the larynx would cause the patient to scream in pain, proving to him that he could indeed speak.

Yealland, who went on to write a book about the patients he allegedly cured, was fervent about his technique; he wrote as "an evangelist grappling with evil, driving the devils from his patient's body."[35] In this, he was no different than Freud, for whom shell shock, reframed as traumatic wartime neurosis, was important only because the condition, as he understood it, validated the psychoanalytic the-ory of peacetime neurosis. "German war medicine has taken the bait" was his self-serving response to a brief pamphlet advocating a mod-ified cathartic approach to shell shock that sought to retrieve from the unconscious the patient's underlying "fixed idea."[36]

The nurses were far removed from such arcana. Theirs was a therapeutic pragmatism of time and place, and it pertained to shell-shocked soldiers no less than soldiers struggling to accept permanent disablement or imminent death. Patients with "functional" symp-toms—symptoms without an apparent anatomical or physiological basis—could be lumped together as shell shock cases for organiza-tional purposes. But the nurses understood they were dealing with wounded soldiers whose conditions often improved over time through human connection with the nurses, acceptance by their wounded comrades, and the containing structure of the hospital ward, which, for all its deprivations, provided many of the shell shocked with an early form of milieu therapy.

• • •

With the shell shocked, the therapeutic gift of the World War I nurses resided less in their ability to empathize than in their acceptance of the fact that their patients had experienced horrors that need not, indeed *could* not, be empathized with. Their duty, their calling, was simply to stay with these soldiers in an accepting manner that coaxed them toward commonality among the wounded. There was nothing here of Yealland-type reeducation. Yealland sought to persuade the shell shocked by logical argument that their condition was not all that serious, that their manifestly physical symptoms were purely mental. Electric shock was a concession to patients' persisting belief that physical symptoms were "real" and called for physical intervention. If both forms of reeducation were unavailing, then the patient would be isolated, bolstering his "stimulus to recovery" by making his illness "a dreary and unprofitable business, instead of a source of pride and satisfaction."[37]

The nurses' approach was diametrically opposite. They sought to cultivate shell-shocked patients' self-acceptance within a community of fellow sufferers, mental and physical. They wanted the shell shocked to arrive at their own sense that their symptoms, fueled by an underlying terror, were not only understandable but unexceptional, and well within the realm of remedial nursing care. In this sense—in the sense of a daily willingness to be with these soldiers in all their bodily dysfunction, mental confusion, and florid symptomatic displays—the nurses strove to normalize shell shock for the shell shocked. They bore in mind that the shell shocked, however dithery, shaking, and stammering, were depressed and scared "only at times." Otherwise, continued Dorothea Crewdson, "they are very cheery and willing." Mary Stollard, a British nurse working with shell-shocked soldiers at a military hospital in Leeds, noted that many of the boys were very sensitive to being incontinent.

> They'd say, "I'm terribly sorry about it, Sister, it's shaken me all over and I can't control it. Just imagine, to wet the bed at my age!" I'd say, "We'll see to that. Don't worry about it." I used to give them a bedpan in the locker beside them and keep it as quiet as possible. Poor fellows, they were so embarrassed—especially the better-class men.[38]

But such embarrassment was a relic of civilian life. The nurses, in both attitude and behavior, worked to convince the shell shocked that they were part of a community of soldiers wounded in the service of their country. Nor did embarrassment have any place among battle-hardened nurses who coped daily with the sensory overload of trench warfare: the overpowering stench of gangrenous infections and decaying flesh; the sight of mutilated soldiers missing arms or legs or faces or portions of torso; the screams of gassed soldiers, blind and on fire and dying in unspeakable pain.

Alongside such things, how off-putting could incontinence be? The shell shocked, no less than the nurses themselves, were soldiers. Soldiers are wounded and scarred in innumerable ways; nurses themselves fell victim to shell shock, even if they were not officially diagnosed as such.[39] Mary Borden wrote of herself as "jerk[ing] like a machine out of order. I was away now, and I seemed to be breaking to pieces." She was sent home as "tired."[40] But then nurses on the front were always tired; they needed and appreciated the rest. It was not so simple for the troops, however. Knowing full well that shell-shocked soldiers declared physically unfit and shipped back home were often subject to stigma and humiliation, Ellen La Motte offered this dismal prognosis for one who had lost the ability to walk and could no longer serve the nation: "For many months he had faced death under the guns, a glorious death. Now he was to face death in another form. Not glorious, *shameful*."[41]

There is this ingrained tendency—an unhappy legacy of the Freudian century—to devalue therapeutic support as superficial, its psychological impact modest and less durable than the kind of hard-won insight that brings repressions and resistances to the light of consciousness. It is such insight that imparts the "Aha" experience and, if emotionally "felt" and "worked through" over time by the patient, results in deep "structural" change in the patient's personality, in this case the traumatized soldier.

This proto-Freudian theory of therapeutic change came to fruition in World War II, when a new generation of barbiturates, especially sodium amytal and sodium pentothal, became the basis of what was termed narcotherapy. In a "cathartic" approach to treatment that hearkened back to Breuer's and Freud's *Studies on Hysteria* of 1895, American army psychiatrists such as John Spiegel, Roy Grinker, and Lawrence Kubie used the new drugs to take GIs back to the battlefield experience nestled in their unconscious that, in the psychoanalytic lingo of the time, had crippled their egos. By re-experiencing battlefield trauma under the reassuring guidance of the psychiatrist, soldiers would experience release of the pent-up aggression that had left them in the grips of a war neurosis.

The nurses of World War I tell a different story with different lessons for the present. Despite preliminary attempts at a Freudian-type talking treatment in select specialty hospitals in Great Britain, such as the Royal Victorian Hospital at Netley, there was no aura of Freudianism in the field and base hospitals of the Allied nurses. Here, once more, it was all about support. But the support more often than not was a support in depth, a support that was stabilizing and mood elevating. There was no possibility of anything more, but neither was there therapeutic warrant for anything else.

The nurses were not alone in espousing this kinder, gentler approach. Among British psychiatrists rehabilitating a select group of shell-shocked soldiers, mainly officers, back in Britain, David Forsyth and Frederick Mott also took a commonsense approach that revolved around patients' comfort, welfare, and amusement. At Mott's Maudsley Hospital, a "beautiful institute outside of London," according to Viets,[42] light and airy wards and day rooms, healthful abundant meals, plenty of recreation, and daily warm or cold spray baths were the order of the day.

The nurses managed to treat thousands of enlisted men this very way, and to do so in CCSs and field hospitals subject to battle rushes and bombings, and that, even during the lulls, provided less than gracious accommodations. Free of the burden of theory-driven directives, they brought to the shell shocked an amalgam of maternalism and scientific authority that normalized mental suffering as an expectable and acceptable vicissitude of battlefield experience. They neither avoided the shell shocked nor infantilized them nor hovered over them in psychoanalytic-type scrutiny. They simply nursed them, thereby conveying the sense that shell shock—whatever its form of expression—signified yet another wartime injury and not the marker of a crippled ego that had collapsed under the weight of a pathogenic fixed idea.

On the Western front, as we have seen, nursing authority partook of medical authority. Within medical staffs that comprised surgeons, graduate nurses, nurse aides, and orderlies, the nurses were the bedside physicians. There were no interns or residents or non-surgeon physicians to manage patients before and after surgery. As clinicians, moreover, the graduate nurses unquestionably stood ahead of the untested medical students who occasionally made their way to field and base hospitals to provide assistance. It is difficult to find testimonies of nurses' effectiveness as bedside counselors with shell-shocked patients, as it was a day-to-day reality of life in the wards. Consider, by way of extrapolation, the testimony of the British nursing aide and gifted writer Vera Brittain.

In the aftermath of a war in which her trials at the front were compounded by the devastating deaths, one after the other, of her fiancé and brother, Brittain found herself in 1920 in the grips of a "horrible delusion" that her face was changing. The delusion devolved into hallucinations and became, in her words, "a permanent, fixed obsession," one that took "full possession of my warped and floundering mind." What was the treatment for this idiosyncratic expression of the shell shock Brittain suffered?

> I have since been told that hallucinations and dreams and insomnia are normal symptoms of over-fatigue and excessive strain, and that, had I consulted an intelligent doctor immediately after the War, I might have been spared the exhausting battle against nervous breakdown which I waged for eighteen months. But no one, least of all myself, realized how near I had drifted to the borderland of craziness.[43]

An intelligent doctor simply conveyed reassurance and thereby drained Brittain's mental abscess. It was no different on the front, where nurses' training and experience, deepened by emotional intelligence, provided a reassurance that was authoritative and often took hold. Such intelligence was at the heart of Mary Stollard's normalizing acceptance of her patient's incontinence. This approach, which deftly provided support in an almost off-handed way, operated among all the wounded, not just the shell shocked. Here is the British nurse Kate Luard, working in a casualty clearing station off the British line in the French commune of Lillers in April 1916. She is at the bedside of a young soldier whose arm was amputated the preceding day:

> A boy in the Surgical, who had his arm amputated yesterday (and was glad to be rid of it), seemed to be worrying about something this morning. It was a perfectly horrible arm, and he hated it. When I said, "But you're glad it's off, aren't you?" he said, "Yes, I am meself, but I'm wonderin' how I'm goin' to keep me family." He had a wife and two children! I told him what splendid new arms soldiers get now, and how everyone would give them the possible jobs, like messengers and Commissionaires, before civilians, and his brow cleared at the rosy visions. I only hope it is true. Is it?[44]

Was implanting a rosy vision of postwar life with a prosthetic arm consistent with the goals of supportive psychotherapy? Perhaps.

Certainly, it cannot be considered an element of what is now termed *dynamic* supportive therapy, with its attentiveness to maladaptive patterns of relating and the defensive "structures" that sustain them. And yet, what more might a supportive therapist have done for a frightened, confused, depressed amputee lying in his hospital bed in a field hospital than Luard did? In the manner of a supportive therapist, Luard succeeded in mobilizing her soldier's adaptive resources in the interest of a therapeutic goal. She succeeded, that is, in conveying a sense of continuity between his life before and after his war-inflicted injury. She used her nursing authority, infused with a healthy dose of maternalism, to replace her patient's fear with hope. In the manner of all effective supportive therapy, she used (rather than interpreted) the transference, here in its maternal guise, as leverage to enable her patient to feel a great deal better in the immediacy of his loss of limb. Yealland's ability to assure shell-shocked patients that he was not only knowledgeable, indeed omniscient, when it came to their "illness," but absolutely confident he could cure them was similarly grounded in the transference. But his goal was not self-acceptance and gradual return to psychological well-being. He wanted to effect swift, if fragile, amelioration of symptoms so that soldiers could be pronounced cured and return to the regiments at the front. There they typically broke down again, to the point that as early as 1915 David Forsyth, among others, argued that those who had suffered what he termed nerve-shock should, with few exceptions, not return to the firing line at all.[45]

And the hopefulness, the rosy vision, is sufficiently moored to reality to be considerably more than a fantasy. The fact is that World War I witnessed the medicalization and standardization of artificial limb manufacture under the control for the first time of orthopedic surgeons. Especially noteworthy were the advances in prosthetic technology coming out of the Office of the Secretary of Defense's Artificial Limb Laboratory at Walter Reed Hospital/Army Medical College.[46]

It is true that, despite government appeals to business for preferential treatment, disabled soldiers, amputees among them, had difficulty finding employment in a postwar economy flooded with veterans and a culture freighted with social Darwinism and the view of the disabled as defectives. Still, nurses like Kate Luard, who coaxed patients out of depression with encouraging scenarios about life after the war offered a vision no rosier than that of home front rehabilitation officials who, in the years following the Armistice, continued to deny the permanence and complexity of limb loss.[47] Nurses like Luard used therapeutic leverage to keep the disabled—shell-shocked patients among them—on the playing field and into the next inning of their lives. This was a short-term goal, addressed through direct measures that, presumably repeated in the days to follow, fostered the patient's ability to adapt to his disability as it pertained to his masculine self-esteem and his life after the war. This is of the essence of supportive therapy.[48]

• • •

Back on the American home front, social workers, many of whom initially trained as nurses, continued their turn to "psychiatric social work," which grew out of the social psychiatry of Adolf Meyers and William Alanson White. In early July 1918, while the AEF nurses were soothing their amputees with a gentle vision of normal life following their heroic sacrifices, Smith College, in collaboration with the Boston Psychopathic Hospital, established the nation's first psychiatric training program for social workers. In the hands of Freudian teachers, American social workers learned to redefine casework as a Freudian project in which the worker, now cast as a psychotherapist, served the client, now a patient, by offering objective insights into the latter's personality, the root cause, so they were taught, of his or her environmental struggles. The immediate goal of the program, which was financially supported by the National Committee of Mental Hygiene, was to place these specially trained psychiatric social workers in stateside base hospitals, where they would help psychiatrists shoulder the burden of shell-shocked soldiers coming home at war's end.

While home front social workers rallied around the Freudian banner in anticipation of returning shell-shocked doughboys, the AEF nurses on the Western front, no more concerned with techniques of engagement than with theories of shell shock, simply stayed the course—supportively. They supported their patients through words, actions, and special accommodations, even if the latter simply meant allowing them to dither on about mates blown to bits or wounded and never brought in. They realized, in a manner America's homegrown Freudians rarely did, the pathogenic self-sufficiency of wartime trauma, of scenes "burnt into their brains,"[49] as a ground for the plentiful and varied symptoms of shell shock.

Can we imagine the psychophysical impact of seeing a comrade literally blown to bits? Or for the nurses, of greeting a convoy, like the young Canadian nurse Clare Gass, and realizing that some casualties would be "so much better dead"—a "young lad with eyes and nose all gone—one blur of mangled flesh" and lads with "heads shattered to pieces."[50] Or finally rushing outside the hospital after a night time bombing raid to discuss the damage wrought by an enormous explosion, only to discover this "unforgettable sight."

> Against the blood red sky of sunrise stood a tree which had spread its bare branches over one of the barracks. For a moment I could think of nothing but a Christmas tree: the building had disappeared and the barren branches had blossomed horribly with fragments of human bodies, arms and legs, bits of bedding, furniture, and hospital equipment.[51]

Such was the experience of Oregonian Shirley Millard, working out of a French evacuation hospital just days after the beginning of the final German offensive in the spring of 1918. These and countless other examples suggest the suprahuman might of the shocks the nurses endured. In their diaries they record scenes more suggestive of the uncanny than of nervous shock in its usual sense. The nurses, no less than combatants, typically fell victim to shell shock not because of the concussive impact of shell explosions, which may or may not have caused microscopic lesions in their brains.[52] For the nurses, nervous collapse, which for the soldiers was always labeled shell shock, often followed scenes of devastation of biblical proportion—scenes that simply could not be assimilated into their sense of self, personal, professional, spiritual, or otherwise. No doubt many succumbed to the cumulative stress of prolonged exposure to what Kate Luard and others termed the "wreckage" of battle wounded. But the instances of shell shock still capable of burning into brains are not those of escalating stress reactions but of instantaneous breakdown before the Horrific.

The Horrific amounts to more than blood and gore. It begins where loss of limb segues into bodily fragmentation. The nurses write of scenes in which explosions do not even leave the remains of identifiable human beings, but only the residue of what were once whole organisms. The scenes, in turn, give rise to recurrent images of "bits" and "pieces" in the nurses' diaries and letters.

The bits and pieces arise in various contexts, but among nurses taking casualties right off the front, they are never far away. There are the bits and pieces dug out of wounds deep and shallow in the service of healing. A nurse writes her mother of washing wounds "huge and ghastly" and then "digging about for bits of shrapnel" or of extracting "bits of cloth and fragments of metal, sometimes at a terrifying depth."[53] Another confronts a patient who, on top of other no less ghastly wounds, has been "pelleted" over his face and body with "small bits of shrapnel, cloth and mud being driven into each tiny wound." "Day by day," she continues, "little bits of shrapnel were dug out till we had cleaned up the whole surface of his body."[54]

Nurses learn of the Horrific second hand. They write of patients who perseverate about "mates who were blown to bits," of returning to find their own officer "blown to bits—a leg in one place, his body in another."[55] A nurse visits a dental ward that reconstructs faces and jaws and cannot "believe it possible to make anything human out of some of the pieces of faces that were left."[56]

And of course they confront the bits and pieces first hand. A nurse stands before "heads shattered to pieces or limbs hanging by a thread of tendons."[57] Another compares her experience to a person standing on the beach, "at whose feet pieces of wreck and corpses are thrown up by the tide."[58] After the bombing of the 58th Scottish Hospital in the fall of 1917, Beatrice Hopkinson watches hospital orderlies "stoop over bunches of twigs in various places and picked up something, putting it into the sheet. They were the arms and legs and other pieces of the patients that had been bombed and blown right out into the park."[59] The orderlies are the forefathers of contemporary army specialists in "mortuary affairs" who retrieve and bag the body parts and liquefied innards of America's fallen soldiers in Afghanistan.[60]

This imagery, so unassimilable as to be ghoulish, reminds us what it meant to be shocked into dysfunction or breakdown during the Great War. Often enough, the bits and pieces signify scenes in which there was no possibility of warding off "unutterable woe" by "saving bits from the wreckage," to recur to the words of the American nurse Kate Norman Derr.[61] Rather, they are scenes in which "saving bits" has been transmuted, darkly, into retrieving bits and pieces of bodies.

Off the battlefield the nurses experienced another version of the Horrific: recurrent scenes of soldiers' dying before their eyes amid blood and gore and dismemberment because the bits and pieces of their bodies could not be surgically reassembled. This is not "shell" shock, but existential shock that, in the psychological lexicon of the psychoanalyst Heinz Kohut, blows apart the cohesive self and the sense of secure groundedness in the world that derives from it.[62] Let one example stand for the many that go unrecorded. It comes from Dorothea Crewdson, a volunteer nurse working at a stationary hospital in Étaples during the final German offensive in May 1918. She writes of another nurse, a W. A. Brampton, of whom nothing is known:

> Poor Brampton must have had a dreadful time and now is suffering from definite shell shock and over in Sick Sisters being looked after. Her two front tanks looked simply terrible the next morning. The floor was smeared with pools of gore and nearly every bed had its gruesome horrible mark—the mattresses all torn and things tossed about everywhere—the whole place a perfect wreck.[63]

6

Plague

"The boys are dying like flies."[1]

Influenza. The Plague. The Great Pandemic of 1918. The Spanish flu, which, as best we can determine, originated not in Spain but in Camp Funston in northeastern Kansas and Camp Oglethorpe in northwestern Georgia in March and April 1918. From there it spread to other army camps, then to France via troops disembarking at Brest, then to the rest of Europe, then to the rest the world. By the time the epidemic had passed, world population was reduced by 50 to 100 million, or from 3 percent to 5 percent.[2]

During 1918 and 1919, 47 percent of all deaths in the United States were from influenza and its complications, with over 675,000 deaths in all. The first wave of the disease in the spring of 1918 was relatively mild, as the virus learned to adapt to humans via passage from person to person. But the second wave, which began in August, was deadly. Philadelphia officials, like municipal officials elsewhere, made light of the looming epidemic and foolishly refused to cancel a Liberty Loan Parade scheduled for September 28. Within three days, every hospital bed in the city's 31 hospitals was filled; within 10 days the pandemic exploded to hundreds of thousands ill, with hundreds of deaths each day. The sick by then had spilled over into emergency hospitals quickly set up in all the city's state armories and many of its parish houses. By October 12, 4,500 Philadelphians had died from the flu; a few weeks later the total was nearly 11,000. Neighboring New York City lost over 21,000 during the same period.[3]

One characteristic of the Spanish flu was that, unlike typical influenza, it targeted younger victims, aged 20–40. The fault was

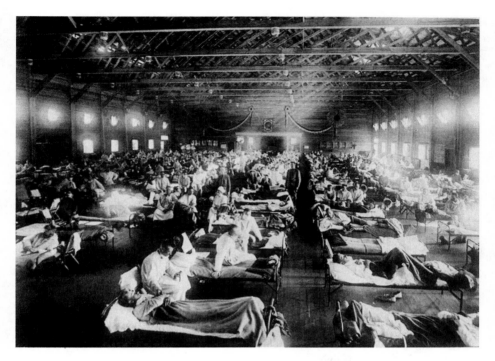

The influenza ward at Camp Funston, Kansas, 1918, probable source of the flu pandemic in the United States.

in their very youth, as their immune systems mounted a massive response to the virus, filling their lungs with so much fluid and debris that the exchange of oxygen became difficult and then impossible. Victims lapsed into unconsciousness and drowned on their own internal secretions. Others remained alive long enough to have bacteria swarm into their compromised lungs and compound viral infection with bacterial pneumonia; when pneumonia set in, the chance of recovery was no greater than 50 percent.

The American Expeditionary Force (AEF) consisted of healthy young men. New recruits lacked immunity to common camp diseases, much less to the deadly Spanish Flu. Influenza hit them hard. Many were already stricken when they boarded transport ships, and many more (about nine percent of Europe-bound troops) contracted flu during the voyage. The USS *Leviathan* was the ne plus ultra. The ship set sail from New York Harbor on September 29, 1918, bound for Brest with 11,000 troops onboard. Prior to disembarking, army inspectors had boarded and removed 100 soldiers with flu symptoms; they then stationed 432 MPs onboard to enforce strict quarantine among the troops. Neither measure was effective. Within one day, 700 men had fallen ill, and, two days later, according to one Navy report, "an inferno raged aboard." On arriving in Brest, 2,000 of the troops on board were stricken. Hundreds died at base hospitals within a matter of days in addition to those buried at sea.[4]

On the home front, things grew desperate in army training camps and cantonments. In Massachusetts's overcrowded encampment in Devon, influenza struck down roughly a third of the 17,000 soldiers in training in September and October; almost 800 of them would die. Nationally, it was the first and only time the number of seriously ill soldiers exceeded the military's total hospital capacity; the army had to take over barracks and use them as hospitals. It was no better overseas, where the virus, imported by survivors of "death ships" like the *Leviathan*, took advantage of the horrific conditions of trench warfare to evolve into its lethal form. By the U.S. War Department's own reckoning, the flu eventually sickened 26 percent of the AEF—over a million men, of whom 340,000 were hospitalized—and accounted for 82 percent of the army's total deaths from disease. During the week of October 4 alone, the army reported 5,160 deaths in its stateside training camps.[5]

The serious shortage of nurses to care for stricken soldiers spurred the American Red Cross to action. It struggled to ship out the 1,000 nurses a week requested by the army. On the home front, it set aside its policy of racial exclusion and enrolled 18 African American nurses for "special service." In early December, two emergency detachments of nurses of color set out for army hospitals at Camp Sherman in Ohio and Camp Grant in Illinois, respectively. There they were assigned to general wards filled with white soldiers. To the surprise of skeptical white chief nurses, their service was exemplary, whatever the drudgery assigned them.[6] Tragically, these 18 nurses, who arrived at their Camps after the Armistice had been signed, represented the sum total of more than 1,800 Red Cross-certified African American nurses called to duty. Even the influenza epidemic, with its overwhelming need for nurses at home and abroad, could not overcome the entrenched racism of the American army and navy.

•   •   •

The story of the pandemic of 1918 is the story of modern medicine not yet modern enough to understand how viruses cause infection at the cellular level. Researchers of the time were bacteriologists but not yet virologists. In 1884, the French microbiologist Charles Chamberland invented a filter with pores smaller than bacteria. This made it possible to pass a solution containing bacteria through the filter and end up with a solution or "filtrate" that was bacteria-free. In 1897, the German bacteriologist Friedrich Loeffler passed the blood of an animal with hoof-and-mouth through the Chamberland filter, only to discover that the filtrate still caused the disease in healthy animals. Two years later, Walter Reed discovered the yellow fever virus in this same manner.

And this is where matters stood at the outbreak of the pandemic of 1918. Given the absence of an operational understanding of viruses—of their structure; of how they invaded and infected cells; even of whether they were liquid or particle in nature—researchers played to the strength of their time: the ability to link specific bacteria to specific illnesses. Understandably, then, the researchers of 1918 searched for a bacteriological culprit for the Spanish Flu—and with good reason. This made eminently good sense to them. It was only a generation earlier, in 1884, that Robert Koch had isolated the bacteria—cholera vibrio—that caused cholera.[7] The following year, Louis Pasteur successfully inoculated 9- and 15-year-old French boys against rabies. And six years later, in 1891, Koch published his paper on tuberculin, and Behring and Kitasato published their paper on tetanus antitoxin that launched the science of serology. Behring published his second paper on diphtheria antitoxin the same year, and when the antitoxin became commercially availability in 1894, the era of "specific immunology" had begun.[8] More than a decade later, in 1908, following an International Tuberculosis Congress held in Washington, the U.S. implemented its agenda for controlling infectious disease, including the universal pasteurization of milk.[9]

But what kind of infectious agent brought on the plague of 1918? In the face of the influenza virus, curative medicine was helpless. There were no antibiotics to combat the bacterial pneumonia that followed viral infection and, researchers now believe, caused far more deaths than the virus itself.[10] Nor could the medicine of 1918 effectively combat respiratory failure, another frequent and severe complication of the viral infection; that medical battle would only be won with the maturing of intensive care units and mechanical ventilators after 1952. Finally, the medicine of 1918 did not permit monitoring of the cardiac complications that usually accompanied severe cases of influenza and were another frequent cause of death.

An arsenal of effective medications to combat any and all such complications would become available during World War II and the decade thereafter. But in 1918 there was little other than supportive care. Vasopressors to increase blood pressure and cardiac inotropes to increase the heart's muscular contractions all lay in the future. Nothing in the toolbox of bacteriology in 1918 could alter the course of the infection or enable physicians to cope effectively with the systemic breakdown that often followed in its wake. Nor, to close the circle, did researchers even know what they were combatting. Only in 1934, when a new flu epidemic raged in Puerto Rico, would Thomas Francis of the Rockefeller Institute, utilizing a technique for viral transmission in animals developed by his colleague Richard Shope, isolate the Type A influenza virus.

• • •

So the warring armies of 1918 were hit hard by the flu, and there was no vaccine to halt its spread and no antiviral therapy to kill the virus among the stricken. There was only nursing care, pushed to its limit by the nurses and nursing aides of the AEF and International Red Cross. Self-evidently, in their prolonged and intimate ministrations to infected soldiers, nurses too contracted the virus, became ill, and occasionally died. During the initially mild phase of the epidemic in the spring of 1918, overseas nurses were content to add flu to the list of maladies that made their lives harder and occasionally took them off the frontlines of ward duty. Being bedridden was simply a vicissitude of the job, a cost of the business of being a combat nurse. "It's not that I mind being in bed," wrote Helen Boylston in February 1918. "I don't even mind having flu and trench fever." Two months later, she recorded that the flu was back again, "and everybody has it, including me. I've run a temperature of one hundred and two for three days, can hardly breathe, and have to sleep on four pillows at night." But she kept her suffering to herself and soldiered on: "But I'm not talking about it, because I don't want to be sent to Villa Tino [for rest and treatment]." At the end of June, Edith Appleton, a British nurse based in Le Tréport, France, wrote of "a very virulent form of influenza spreading like wildfire among the hospitals and ours is nearly full up with them, all with temperatures of anything up to 104 or 105." But, even in the face of such high fevers, Appleton was clueless as to the meaning of the epidemic, including the prognosis of those severely infected. "The good thing," she added hopefully but speciously, "is it is usually over in a week."[11]

By September 1918, most nurses appreciated the seriousness of the flu; it was the "bugbear" in the otherwise heartening war news then coming in.[12] But not all of them. More specifically, some nurses still failed to apprehend that the influenza now attacking soldiers, doctors, and nurses alike was not the milder, often trifling, flu of pre–1918 or even the nonlethal, first wave of epidemic flu of the preceding spring. For Milwaukee's Helen Bulovsky, writing home from Base Hospital 22 at Beau Desert in Southwest France, it was simply a matter of "many of the girls" getting sick with "something like grippe."

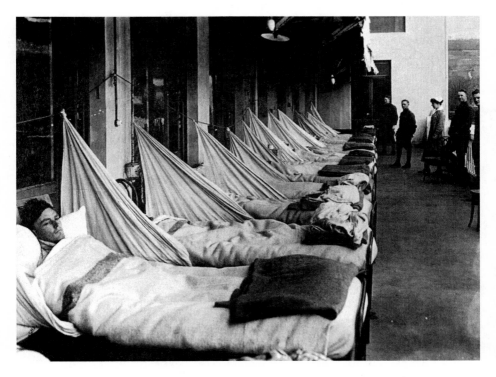

Influenza ward in an American Hospital in France, 1918. Sheet dividers, commonly used, provide token "isolation" of patients.

Nora Saltonstall, an upper-class Bostonian who served in a military ambulance (*autochir*) unit and, near war's end, as a nursing aide, was among the latter. In letters to family members of mid–September, she breezily dismissed the flu as a "local epidemic" that did not leave victims "seriously sick."[13]

Saltonstall could not have been more wrong. When the influenza struck in full force in the fall of 1918, the nurses, whatever their understanding of it or resolve to carry on despite it, were not spared. In the U.S., 127 army nurses died from flu, and an untold number, probably another 100, died in Europe. Katherine Magrath, the chief nurse of U.S. Base Hospital 68 in Nièvre in central France, buried 12 of her nurses in a single month. After each funeral, she avoided looking at the faces of her surviving nurses lest she wonder "which would be the next to be absent from the dismal scene."[14]

Unable to combat the flu at its source, the nurses did what they had grown accustomed to doing for the desperately ill: They bore witness to suffering and tried to ease it. And their witnessing, which could last anywhere from a few hours to a few months, was different from that of the doctors. It included the sensory realities of bodily decay among dying soldiers. The nurses' reminiscences record the sensory experience of hands-on care of those with terminal infections. Influenza cases had swamped the nurses, wrote Shirley Millard at the beginning of April 1918. And the soldiers, "when they die, as about half of them do, they turn a ghastly dark gray and are taken out at once and cremated." Forty of 160 patients had the flu, and the staff was coming down with it. So reported Hoosier nurse Maude Essig from Base Hospital 32 in the French resort town of Contrexéville in November. "The odors," she added, "are bad." Another American nurse, Mary Dobson, destined for Base Hospital 63 in Savenay, treated influenza victims in the infirmary of the troopship during her crossing of late September. She recalled that "the odor was terrible in that ship's infirmary—I never smelt anything like it before or since. It was awful, because there was poison in this virus."[15] Back on the home front, a student nurse on hospital duty recalled desperately ill flu patients, frequently comatose, arriving in the emergency room, "their faces and nails as blue as huckleberries."[16]

Treatment of the flu-ridden called forth everything of a palliative nature in the nurses' toolbox. They quickly learned the course of the illness and took from the toolbox everything they had that might strengthen the heart, ease respiration, bring down fevers, and attenuate suffering. If they could not subdue the virus, they might, with luck, outmaneuver it, keeping gravely ill patients alive long enough for their immune systems to rally and join the struggle. It was a war of logistics that ceded superior strength to the enemy. During the early days of the pandemic, Beatrice Hopkinson wrote of how flu-ridden patients were stripped of their clothing in one tent, bathed in disinfectant and then distributed among different wards. But disinfectants did no good. Two different injectable serums—antitoxins derived from the fluid serum of the blood of immune animals—were made available to the nurses, but neither helped. The nurses were left with milk diets, alcohol rubs, expectorants, cardiac stimulants, cough syrups, and always aspirin. Whatever the routine, the seriously ill patients still died from pneumonia, often within a few days.[17]

Palliation was still important, as much for the nurses as the patients. It entailed a protocol, and with the protocol came a glimmer of hope. For desperately ill soldiers, too, the protocol provided a sense of being cared for by nurses who were not only mothers and sisters but also representatives of the scientific medicine of the time. Contrast this with the efforts of Civil War nurses to ease suffering. For them palliation did not open to a protocol. Yes, they could prepare poultices, serve milk toast, and sit with and read to the ill and wounded, all enveloped in a willingness to sacrifice vouchsafed by religion. With the dying especially, the willingness to sacrifice tended to supplant nursing initiatives altogether. Standing before a soldier with shattered knees who simply lay in bed in agony, the Confederate nurse Kate Cumming simply observed that she "would sacrifice almost anything to palliate his pain."[18]

Still, the best of the Civil War nurses did not stop with a predisposition to self-sacrifice; they became combative defenders of the well-being of "our poor boys," assuming multiple roles of wound dressers, administrators, transport organizers, and comforters of the dying. Wounded soldiers derived inestimable benefit from such women, especially those from their home states whose charge, like that of Maine's Sarah Smith Sampson, was "to try to calm the confusion, to stop some agony."[19] But there was nothing of modern, or even proto-modern nursing care in these efforts.

There was much more for trained nurses and aides to do in the Great War, even in the context of palliation. Wards were kept at an "even temperature" and patients were kept warm and given fluids, placed on milk diets, and given Bovril with milk if they could hold anything down.[20] Primitive blood transfusions, cupping to relieve congestion, giving the fevered alcohol baths or wrapping them in cold wet sheets[21]—all were given a try. With flu victims, the goal was to bring down high fevers and to keep hearts beating and lungs exchanging oxygen and carbon dioxide. The goal invited improvisatory nursing, heroic nursing that squeezed everything possible out of the toolbox at hand. Here, for example, is how nurses coped with a signal corps switchboard operator—one of the first "Hello Girls"—stricken with influenza on board the transport ship *Olympic* in September 1918:

> Risking their own lives, nurses placed warm mustard packs on her chest to dilate the capillaries, stimulate her nervous system, and help her cough up the mucus that could drown her. They aspirated her lungs, sponged her body with alcohol, applied camphorated oil every hour, gave her salt-solution enemas, and spoon-fed her concoctions of milk, eggs, and whiskey. The first week, Conroy received four hypodermic injections of digitalis to control her pulse and strengthen her heartbeat.[22]

This is palliation with a vengeance. None of these ministrations attacked the virus, but they kept Conroy alive, and after 17 days her fever finally broke. She, along with the nurses who saved her, proceeded on to France and the war.

In 1916, prior to the epidemic, nurses who began to feel "influenza-ish" might take brisk walks, perhaps a "good hot mustard bath." But when they took ill after the epidemic set in, they resorted to large doses of quinine and aspirin, along with the occasional "stiff dose of whiskey" to keep going.[23] By the fall of 1918, nurses no longer jested about their misery. Their wards had become "influenza departments," and the healthy among them wondered how long they could resist infection. More often than not, nurses became patients, taking to their beds to await transfer to nearby convalescent homes set aside for them (and referred to colloquially as "Sick Sisters") for treatment and recuperation.[24]

On the home front, student nurses enrolled in the newly established Army School of Nursing discontinued classroom study to nurse patients and sick nurses alike in stateside base hospitals.[25] Students at hospital nursing schools left the classroom to spend long hours on wards overwhelmed with flu patients. One such student, Dorothy Deming, was assigned to the women's flu ward of New York's

Presbyterian Hospital, then a 250-bed facility where 90 graduate and student nurses themselves fell victim to the flu. "Life," she would recall, "was just one long emergency." Nurses on the home front, who worked to the point of exhaustion and assumed medical responsibilities beyond their training, liked to consider themselves soldiers. Deming, for one, considered the nurses at Presbyterian "as truly under fire as though we were with our brothers in the Argonne." Another, Gertrude Peabody, president of Boston's Visiting Nurses Association, averred that her nurses "rendered as noble service as any soldiers in battle."[26]

The equivalence was well-intended but strained. Yes, dedicated nurses on the home front worked long, grueling hours in civilian hospitals, and yes, they rendered exemplary service to their patients, their profession, and their country. But unlike military nurses and aides, their shifts, though exhausting, did come to an end; they were well fed, and they slept on warm, dry beds with mattresses. Their nights were not interrupted by "rushes" of freshly wounded off the battlefield that summoned all nurses, aides, orderlies, and surgeons to battle, often nonstop for up to 48 hours. They were not, in a contemporary idiom, first responders for "the grotesque mutilations of bodies and limbs and faces" that were carried off convoys after major battles, often several hundred at a time, when "bodies stacked or strewn on every surface transformed the hospital into a shadow of the battlefield."[27] Nor, finally, did they tend their flu patients in the kind of chronic discomfort endemic in casualty clearing stations, field hospitals, and general military hospitals, of which Vera Brittain provided a demoralizing listing in 1915: "We all acquired puffy hands, chapped faces, chilblains and swollen ankles, but we seldom actually went sick, somehow managing to remain on duty with colds, bilious attacks, neuralgia, septic fingers, and incipient influenza."[28]

On the Western front, replacement nurses were often unavailable, so AEF nurses labored on despite multiple discomforts that segued into serious illnesses. For many, only physical collapse on the wards could remove them from the second battlefield. Once removed, infected Sisters struggled to return to duty, many without success. Those nurses, like Grace Anderson, who contracted what was termed "slight cases" of flu, did recover and return to duty. Anderson was even able to keep her pregnancy secret during her convalescence. Others, like the Canadian Katherine Wilson, were struck down with

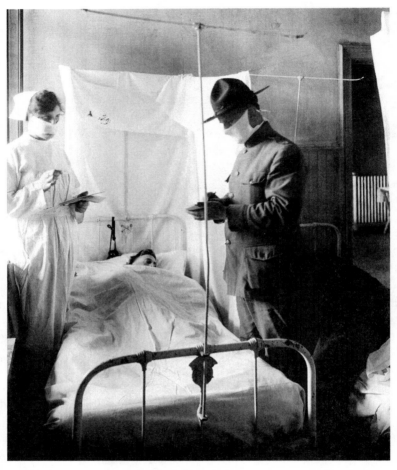

Masked nurse and doctor attend an influenza patient, France, 1918.

virulent influenza "with complications" in November 1916, five months before the first milder wave of the pandemic. After convalescing in England, she returned to Canada for extended leave, only to take her discharge, marry her fiancé, a disabled Canadian infantry officer, and accompany him to Kansas City, Missouri. There the two ran a British-Canadian Recruiting Mission, seeking to persuade Canadians who had crossed over to the United States to avoid military service to return to their country.[29]

♦   ♦   ♦

The flu paid no heed to the Armistice that ended hostilities on November 11, 1918. It raged on in base hospitals and overcrowded embarkation centers, subsiding in intensity in the final month of the year only to return with renewed virulence in the winter of 1919. Any impulse to celebrate the peace dissipated quickly among nurses freighted with the postwar burden of infectious disease. Sent to a newly opened military hospital outside Paris to take charge of medical patients, Elizabeth Weaver, a Red Cross nurse who served with the University of Pennsylvania Unit, offered a less than sanguine assessment. In December 1918, she recorded in her journal, the hospital had 1200 patients and her own ward of 70 including patients with pleurisy (inflammation of the membrane around the lungs), pleurodynia (stabbing chest or abdominal pain), bronchitis, myocarditis (inflammation of the heart muscle), pyrothorax [*sic*] (pus-filled infection of the chest cavity) and TB—in addition to abundant cases of influenza and pneumonia.[30] Reassigned to postwar duty in occupied Germany, she travelled to Coblenz, where she found influenza "raging in the Army of Occupation." On her ward alone, four or five patients a night died, for a total of 52 deaths in three weeks. One of her flu patients, who spiked a fever of 106.4, was in a "raging delirium" and at the point of jumping out the window when Weaver entered the room. "I caught him just in the nick of time," she wrote. "I want the windows protected, for it is absolutely impossible for two people [viz., two nurses] to watch a whole ward full of desperately ill patients & be responsible for same."[31] Assigned night duty in a different ward in March 1919, she watched another 74 patients die, mainly of flu complications, in the course of five weeks.[32]

AEF nurses not part of the Army of Occupation usually remained in base hospitals throughout France and Belgium, serving not only bedridden soldiers but the local populace as well. Then, pooling their efforts with women physicians who served in American Women's Hospitals (AWH) sponsored by the Medical Women's National Association and funded by the American Red Cross, they fanned out from northern France and Belgium to Serbia, the Near East, and even Russia. Working hand in hand with medical colleagues, the nurses established public health programs for civilian populations that had gone without medical, surgical, dental, and nursing care since 1914. Divided into mobile units, AEF nurses and AWH physicians established weekly house call and dispensary routes that took them to battle-scarred villages throughout the regions they served. During the seven months that AWH No. 1 was based in Luzancy in northcentral France, for example, its units made 3,626 house calls to the 20 villages on their regular schedule and to 45 outlying villages as well. In virtually every village, chronic disease management shared center stage with dental and gynecological care. Among the diseases that nurses and physicians continued to battle, typhoid fever and influenza had pride of place.

The same willingness to press on after the Armistice typified units of a rival organization of women physicians and nurses, the Women's Oversea Hospitals (WOH). Whereas most WOH units continued their work with refugees in France after the Armistice, the founding unit organized by Caroline Finley went to Metz, Germany, to treat German prisoners of war, many of whom were bedridden with influenza, in alliance with the French Army of Occupation.[33] At the invitation of the British, a unit of ARC nurses journeyed to a hospital in Jerusalem where, serving under the British Expeditionary Force, they joined local nurses in managing infectious diseases, especially malaria, treating serious wounds via the Dakin-Carrel method, and cleaning and dressing skin grafts.[34]

We have already considered the manner in which nursing care, as implemented by a trained nurse, could become curative by dint of its frequency and intensity, not to mention the bravado with which it was given. Nowhere was this in greater evidence than with the soldiers and civilians stricken with virulent flu in the fall of 1918 and winter of 1919. Nurses in the Allied Expeditionary Force, no less than their sisters-in-arms in the British and Canadian Expeditionary Forces, stayed on and nursed on, no matter the inevitability of patients' death. They warded off resignation and clung to the hope that caring interventions laced with science might at any point turn the tide, if only in the sense of gaining a brief reprieve during which the body's depleted healing resources could rally.

Nurses more than physicians believed in the body's ability to launch counterattacks against ravaging infections that physicians pronounced fatal. Fevers might break. Hearts might return to normal rhythms. Lungs might expel enough infectious matter to resume respiration. And all such things would be sequelae of a nursing strategy of relentless, even desperate, palliation. Surgeons of the Civil War occasionally acknowledged that nursing care, especially when concentrated on a nurse's "special patient," saved lives.[35] But it was the nurses of World War I who, with flu victims especially, elevated this contingency to a modus operandi. Nora Saltonstall, the Bostonian who served in France as, variously, an ambulance driver, auto mechanic, food procurer, and sometime nursing aide, understood the nursing imperative as pushing palliation beyond the zone of physiologically based comfort altogether. In July 1918, she wrote her family of her belief "in having women to nurse them [influenza patients] even if the women are in danger, because the moral effect on the men is beyond belief."[36]

Needless to say, the moral uplift provided by nurses only went so far, and the worst of the influenza patients invariably died. But then so did the worst of the postsurgical patients, the worst of the patients with multiple injuries and multiple amputations, and the worst of the patients exposed to poison gas. It mattered not. Nursing professionals professed an ethic of caring grounded in, but not limited by, the scientific medicine of the time. Standing on the sidelines, Nora Saltonstall knew this only too well. When all else failed, when surgeons and physicians had given up on a patient, nursing care might still become a clinical tipping point that loosened the grasp of the grim reaper. The point was readily conceded by the surgeons. Absent any ability to control the bacterial infestation of densely packed clearing stations and field hospitals that invited secondary infection, they ceded that influenza victims' best hope of recovery rested with nurses.[37]

But what was the basis of this hope? A clean, dry environment in the tradition of late-nineteenth-century sanitary science, improvised expectorants, cough medicines (but not opium), injections of digitalis or nitroglycerin (if either was available) or caffeine or camphorated oil to keep the heart beating, aspirin, phenacetin, quinine, atropine, cocaine, morphine, strychnine—this was the arsenal with which nurses met the enemy. Keep the flu patients dry, warm, hydrated, and as clean and well-nourished as circumstances permit. Aspirate their lungs and use everything in the toolbox to get them to expectorate, inject small amounts of atropine or strychnine or cocaine as stimulants, and give them aspirin, plenty of aspirin. Mother them and console them, and as their end approaches, "stand by them in their last great hour."[38]

In World War I, the "last great hour" was not shrouded in the religiosity of Civil War nursing. There was no celebration, however muted, of soldiers who died sincere and devout Christians. Nor was the pain of loss mitigated by Christian belief in the life to come, as with Louisa May Alcott, for whom "a virtuous and useful life untimely ended is always tragical to those who see not as God sees," or Amanda Akin Sterns, for whom a dying soldier "found rest in that dreamless slumber whose reveille is only heard beyond the grave."[39] The nurses of World War I, standing before the same dying patient, did not, like the Confederate nurse Ada Bacot, beseech God to "grant his sickness may be sanctified to him" in readying his soul for what was to follow.[40] Rather, the vast majority witnessed soldiers' final days bolstered only by duty, the obligation of calling, and the bond of fellowship. Working as neither commissioned nor noncommissioned officers, lacking the authority and security of rank and equal pay, the nurses still bore witness to dying soldiers as comrades-in-arms. And very occasionally, they found, the act of bearing witness, with the simple ministrations it entailed, provided more than they hoped for. Very occasionally the body's immune system would rally, fevers would lessen, pneumonic coughs would abate, and deathly ill soldiers would begin to eat and revive.

For those hit hardest by influenza, the odds were never good and in fact were terrible, but the nurses always gave it their all. It was less what they did than who they were. They were nurses at work; activity was key. Saving "bits from the wreckage," wrote Kate Norman Derr, prevented nurses from being "mastered by the unutterable woe."[41]

•   •   •

The women hospital workers of the Civil War also battled infectious disease, especially malaria, typhoid fever, typhus, and diphtheria. Among midwestern troops who had never been exposed to childhood diseases, they coped with outbreaks of virulent measles, mumps, and chicken pox. And like the nurses of the wars to follow, they tended soldiers suffering the most common and transmittable of infectious diseases: dysentery, which reportedly affected 700 out of 1,000 soldiers and was always accompanied by chronic diarrhea. Inevitably, nurses too succumbed to these diseases. What chance did they have of resisting transmittable typhoid and dysentery when volunteer troops evinced "ungovernable behavior," ignoring orders of where to defecate and when to wash, so that "vast acreages were essentially giant cesspools and garbage dumps"?[42]

The Spanish-American War (SAW) of 1898, even more than the Civil War, was a war of epidemic disease in the temporary camp hospitals of Florida, Georgia, and Long Island and the military hospitals of Cuba and the Philippines. The U.S. Army, which had learned nothing from the Civil War about the central role of trained nurses, entered the war with a skeletal nursing staff of 520 male hospital corpsmen, many of whom were incoming privates with no nursing skills, and 200 male hospital stewards. The call for trained women nurses came quickly in the face of massive infectious illness in the training camps and among soldiers returning from Cuba and Puerto Rico. "Thousands have died from wounds and disease," remarked Nicholas Senn, chief surgeon of the Sixth Army Corps, which saw action in Cuba. "Yellow Fever, dysentery, malaria and typhoid fever have been and continue to be our most formidable enemies." They were "the greatest terrors of camp life."[43] When yellow fever hit Siboney, Cuba in July 1898, the magnitude of the epidemic, and the Army Medical Corps' inability to cope with it, led to the evacuation of the entire Fifth Corps from Cuba to Camp Wikoff at the tip of Long Island, where deaths from both yellow fever and typhoid fever continued to mount.[44]

It was women nurses, many graduates of the hospital training programs that arose in the decade following the Civil War, who were immediately recruited to combat these twin epidemics. Their struggle, as with their predecessors in the Civil War and their successors in World War I, was to nurse on, up to 16 hours a day, without succumbing to systemic infections themselves. Circumstances were not conducive to the latter. Dr. Laura Hughes, superintendent of nurses in the detention hospital of Camp Wikoff, observed that orderlies uncomprehending of the nature of infection and its transmission, were continually emptying the bedpans of typhoid fever victims just outside their tents.[45] At Sternberg Field Hospital in Chickamauga Park, Georgia, 200 nurses made do with three toilets located 500 feet from their sleeping quarters—the slightest of improvements over "vast acreages" covered with feces and garbage surrounding the tent hospitals of Civil War nurses. Nor did the majority of SAW nurses have hot water, or even much cold water; bathing facilities were nonexistent. Along with their patients, they dined on fly-infested salt pork and beans in temperatures of over 100 degrees. Small wonder that many SAW nurses fell victim to malaria; that at least 10 percent of them contracted typhoid fever; and that virtually all the nurses in particular camps came down with a virulent dysentery that plagued many for life.[46]

All war is hell for combatants. Battlefield nurses share in the hell, and it is pointless to compare degrees of privation, misery, and suffering among nurses of different wars; each nurse, like each soldier, has her own story. What then gives the Great Pandemic of 1918 its mystique? Why is it considered by many the ne plus ultra in the long dispiriting list of life-threatening contagious diseases contracted by American soldiers during wars of the nineteenth and twentieth centuries? There is no single answer to the question, but rather a web of interrelated factors that contribute to this sense of singularity. Most obviously, there was the simultaneity with which the virus created mass casualties among warring armies across a broad expanse of world geography. There was also the stunning speed with which it felled its victims. Among the severely infected, influenza often ran its course in a day, and the course almost always ended in death. "The hospital is overrun with flu," reads Helen Boylston's diary entry of October 24, 1918. "We've had it every year, of course, but nothing like this. The boys are dying like flies." In the small wards tended by Beatrice Hopkinson, "it became terrible ... the boys were dying in threes and fours nightly."[47] Among those who did not die like flies but were dying nonetheless, the flu led to a prolonged end-stage over a period of weeks, during which the nurses' toolbox, mined for any possible agent of comfort, became useless to attenuate the suffering of the disease's final victory.

From the standpoint of medicalized nursing care, it is the historical context of the nurses' relative helplessness that comes to the fore. Between the Spanish-American War and World War I, American nurses proceeded along the path to professionalism that began after the Civil War and gained expression in the founding of the first three hospital training schools in 1873. Nurse professionalism was bolstered by the exemplary service of graduate nurses in training camps and military hospitals during the Spanish-American War, the "splendid little war" of 1898. The military took note of the nurses' ability to tolerate heat, flies, and filth and still provide intensive nursing care to soldiers struck down by typhoid and yellow fever. Seeking to ensure the rapid mobilization of graduate nurses in future conflicts, it established the Army Nurse Corps in 1901.

Nurse professionalism made further gains at this time and in the decade to follow. In 1899, in the midst of the Spanish-American War, the Society of Superintendents for Nurses, led by Isabel Hampton and Mary Nutting, initiated postgraduate education for nurses at Teachers College of Columbia University; the first generation of professional nurse educators emerged from this program.[48] Nineteen hundred saw publication of the first issue of the *American Journal of Nursing*, and 1908 saw the organization of African American nurses into the National Association of Colored Graduate Nurses (NACGN), partly to combat a racist system of dual state registration in southern states.[49] A year later in 1909 the University of Minnesota established the first university-based school of nursing in the country. In the same year, nurse home visits (i.e., house calls) received the imprimatur of the Metropolitan Life Insurance Company, which began paying nurses from Lillian Wald's Henry Street Settlement $.50 per visit to policy holders of the "industrial" (i.e., working) classes. Finally, establishment of the federal Children's Bureau within the Department of Labor in 1912 further elevated the role of professional nursing care, especially the maternal and infancy care provided by public health nurses.

The nurses of the Great War were beneficiaries of these developments, and they embraced a role that did not consign them to providing tea and sympathy in the form of additional blankets, better nutrition, sponge baths, cooling compresses, and letter writing. Rather, their role was interventionist in a nascently modern way. They were expected, that is, to do medically necessary things to aid in the stabilization, treatment, and recovery of the wounded and the ill. We have considered many of these activities and interventions in preceding chapters: nurses administering anesthesia and assisting in major surgery; nurses performing bedside surgery on their own and initiating procedures such as Dakin-Carrel irrigation; nurses improvising aids to respiration and various orthopedic devices to immobilize major fractures. In the casualty clearing stations and field hospitals of France and Belgium, nurses were the triage officers, determining which incoming patients required emergency interventions, which immediate transfer to surgical huts, and then, in recovery, which most required postsurgical nursing care, including procedural interventions.

To be sure, comfort care was an important component of World War I nursing. But unlike Civil War nurses and much more so than

SAW nurses, the World War I nurses provided comfort care as an adjunct to medicalized caregiving that strove to be scientific. Only in the Great War, that is, did they become true partners in medical and surgical care. Civil War nurses may have, in the words of Louisa May Alcott, laid back on the shelf their "carefully prepared meekness" and entered the fray. But, in tent hospitals off the battlefield, the fray they entered and the battles they fought had more to do with camp corruption and patient abuse than the fight to save lives in medically salient ways. In the Confederacy, lady nurses of elevated social standing—South Carolina's Ada Bacot is one example—often arrived at general hospitals with a slave in tow and confined their hospital work to the conventional woman's sphere, which meant the kitchen and the laundry. The Union nurse Cornelia Hancock wrote of dressing wounds in Fredericksburg after the Battle of the Wilderness, but only because "there was no food but hard tack to give the men" and she had nothing else to do. For the lady nurses of the Civil War, food always came first.[50] Certainly SAW nurses risked their lives nursing typhoid and yellow fever victims in camps overwhelmed by these epidemics. But their nursing ministrations—except as initiated by the handful of women physicians who served as chief nurses[51]—were essentially custodial in nature.

The forward-looking aspect of World War I nursing hardly tarnishes the heroism of nurses in earlier wars; rather it underscores the manner in which nursing care during the Great War anticipates modern nursing practice. Civil War and SAW nurses were not simply nurses, trained or otherwise, but women helpmates for whom the ethic of Florence Nightingale was at the heart of their endeavor. Unsurprisingly, surgeons and military officers alike sought out nurses for whom this ethic was most intrinsic to their identity: the Nursing Sisters of the Catholic Orders, especially the Daughters of Charity, for whom self-discipline, selfless devotion to others, and absolute obedience to superiors were religious imperatives. Most desirable of all were Catholic Sisters whose religious calling was fortified by nurse training. It was the scientific training and curative, or at least remedial, expectations of the Great War nurses and doctors that amplified the horror of the Great Plague and, in retrospect, heighten its singularity.

•   •   •

In the final months of World War I everything changed. Surrounded by flu patients dying like flies, often in unrelievable agony, many nurses did feel the situation hopeless; certainly, they felt helpless to alter the disease's course or even to attenuate its symptoms with the respiratory aids, cardiac stimulants, and analgesics at hand. This helplessness was difficult to bear precisely because it was out of sync with their hard-won identities as professional caregivers. They expected not merely to cope, but to cope in ways that were scientifically informed and medically consequential. This meant availing themselves of everything in their toolbox and, typically in the absence of doctors, using these tools to maximum effect, often in creative, problem-solving ways. With the sickest of the influenza patients, this expectation was dashed. To return full circle, the microbiology of 1918 and the serum therapies that derived from it were impotent in the face of a virus whose understanding fell to virologists of the next generation.

Nurses, no less than physicians, could not understand what was simply not understandable. This is because, like all scientific caregivers, they operated within a paradigm that was epistemologically constraining.[52] Like all scientific paradigms, this one determined both the type of questions that could be asked and the type of answers that could be sought. The nurses of World War I, no less than the surgeons alongside whom they worked, could only pose certain questions about the nature of infectious disease—its agent, its mode of action, its transmission, and its treatment. The assumptions with which they approached such theoretical and clinical matters were those of Pasteur, Koch, Kitasato, Shiga, von Bering, and others who ushered in the glory era of late-nineteenth-century bacteriology. Its signal achievements included the identification of specific bacteria responsible for specific illnesses—the cholera vibrio, the tubercle bacillus, the Corynebacterium diphtheriae (or Klebs-Löffler bacillus), and the bacillus dysenterie. And it made great progress on other fronts. At the time of the Great War, an effective typhoid vaccine existed and the technology to preserve it and ship it overseas was in place. Even before America's entry into the war, the Hygienic Laboratory of the Public Health Service had isolated organisms from epidemic meningitis, developed tetanus antitoxin, and improved Almroth Wright's anti-typhoid vaccine of 1897.[53] But the late-nineteenth century paradigm, for all its stunning achievements, could not yield an answer to epidemic killer flu.

By World War I cracks had begun to appear in the paradigmatic structure of nineteenth-century bacteriology—Alexander's Fleming's finding of 1915 that antiseptics were not only useless but harmful in the treatment of infected wounds is one example.[54] But the paradigm was able to contain the anomalies that arose. Even at the height of the epidemic, the nurses shared the bacteriologists' belief that germ theory as it then existed would rise to the occasion and provide new serums effective against the flu. But they were wrong. "None of the Doctors seem to know much about it but they think it is Streptococi [*sic*] pneumonia," Alice O'Brien wrote her parents from Paris in late October 1918. "Everyone has been warned to take precautions against it, gargling with antiseptic, etc., and the authorities are in hopes of getting it under control before long."[55] But the flu was not a bacterial pneumonia, even though bacterial pneumonia invariably followed those with severe infections. Nor was it caused by the *Bacillus influenzae* discovered by the German bacteriologist Richard Pfeiffer in 1892, another causal candidate considered and rejected by bacteriologists of the time. Inevitably, the serums derived from these bacteria were ineffective; the results from their use, reported the American-trained Canadian nurse Alice Isaacson, simply "not good."[56]

It followed that precautions rooted in late nineteenth-century bacteriology were of virtually no help. The flu virus was not a bacteria of any kind, so it was not susceptible to the preventive measures intrinsic to public health campaigns waged against bacterial invaders. Gargling with antiseptics, covering the mouth when sneezing or coughing, refraining from spitting, partially separating ward beds with sheets, even placing patients in individual canvas tents—all such measures, widely circulated in placards and posters of the time, were largely useless against the virus.

Even the gauze masks of the time, porous as they were, accomplished very little.[57] Occasionally a nurse jettisoned bacteriological thinking altogether; Helen Bukovsky, for example, suggested that nurses who remained unbothered by the flu had acquired resistance because "we have been well toughened by living in tents."[58]

So the graduate nurses of World War I, whose training was informed by scientific medicine of the time, seized on the vestiges of nineteenth-century sanitary science to combat the flu. But the influenza ran its course anyway. The nurses brought science to bear in their efforts to contain the Great Epidemic, but it was science constrained by a paradigm that was inadequate to the task. In 1918 this was the bacteriologist's quandary and the nurses' special hell. In 1918 hell approached them from all directions. It was expressed in the war itself, given that "one is never equipped nor prepared for such Hellishness." Nurses such as Alice O'Brien gleaned hell especially in the faces of soldiers returning from gas attacks. But it was the nurses' helplessness before the influenza virus—a natural catastrophe in the midst of a man-made disaster—that brought them to hell's portal, since, among the severely infected it denied them even the possibility of comfort care, whether restorative or simply soothing. "It is dreadful to be impotent," wrote a nurse from her Belgian field hospital, "to stand by grievously stricken men it is impossible to help, to see the death-sweat gathering on young faces, to have no means of easing their last moments. This is the nearest to Hell I have yet been."[59]

To be sure, this impotence before the grievously stricken was not limited to dying influenza patients of 1918. It pertained to soldiers with massive battlefield injuries beyond surgical repair and to those blinded and burning up with poison gas. The impotence before flu victims was arguably greater because of the scope of the epidemic, the terrifying speed with which healthy soldiers were transformed into dying ones, and the absence of any visible markers of war-related injury. Victims of the flu simply became very sick and died. The scientifically trained minds of the World War I nurses could understand what was wrong, but their eyes could not see it in a manner that might have contained it and eased their sense of helplessness. It was analogous to soldiers who, lying deep in their trenches, knew they were under assault but were helpless against an unseen enemy. This particular hell was captured by the young poet Alan Seeger, an American volunteer serving in the trenches with French compatriots. In a letter to the *New York Sun* published on December 8, 1914, he informed his countrymen that the role of the "poor common soldier" in trench warfare was "anything but romantic":

> His role is simply to dig himself a hole in the ground and to keep hidden in it as tightly as possible. Continually under the fire of the opposing batteries, he is yet never allowed to get a glimpse of the enemy. Exposed to all the dangers of war, but with none of its enthusiasms or splendid *élan*, he is condemned to sit like an animal in its burrow and hear the shells whistle over his head and take their little daily toll from his comrades.

For the soldiers on the front, this enforced passivity before the enemy was the main thing. For the wounded, it often persisted in hospitals. "It must be an uncomfortable feeling," wrote Shirley Millard in April 1918, "for the men to lie helpless in bed, with arms strapped up or down fastened tightly to a frame, or legs in casts, aware that directly over their heads are enemy planes loaded with bombs."[60] Uncomfortable indeed. The nurses who confronted the ravages of the Great Pandemic faced their own variants of enforced passivity, of ocular and experiential blindness to the enemy within. At its peak in the fall of 1918, the pandemic threatened to crack the foundation of their self-consciousness as partners in scientifically informed caregiving. No less importantly, among those severely infected, it provided little time or opportunity for nurses to slip into their traditional role of maternal comforters. The nurses who labored on, often ill themselves, "nursing through"[61] profound despondency at how little they could do, were perhaps ironically beacons of modernity. Using their toolbox to no great avail while awaiting new and effective serums, they crossed the Rubicon into a medical age of unsettled modernity.

• • •

The nurses' struggle to contain catastrophic infectious disease with the ineffectual remedies at hand is another aspect of the singularity of the Great Pandemic, both in context and in retrospect. It showed that medicine could be scientific and still fail to meet the emergency at hand. This reality heralded an age in which scientific medicine and infectious disease continuously leapfrogged ahead of one another, with laboratory researchers conquering one infectious disease only to confront a more treatment-resistant one around the corner.

The process antedated the Great War by only several years. The arsenic compound Salvarsan, the first proto-antibiotic, was released to the public at the very end of 1910. It was effective with the spirochetes that caused syphilis, but its toxicity led to side effects that many found worse than the infection. The sulfa drugs of the mid–1930s were curative with the streptococcal bacteria that caused sore throats, erysipelas, and puerperal (childbirth) infections, but left untouched the gram-positive bacteria that caused deadly staphylococcal infections. Effective treatment of the latter awaited the purification of penicillin in the 1940s, which then replaced Salvarsan-derivatives in the treatment of syphilis; it was equally effective against gonorrhea bacilli. But penicillin proved ineffective against the bacteria that caused tuberculosis (mycobacterium tuberculosis), which then yielded to streptomycin and aminosalicylate sodium (PAS), simultaneously discovered several years later.

But streptomycin and PAS, like penicillin, had no effect on viruses, including the one that caused the influenza pandemic of 1918. The researchers leapfrogged ahead in 1957, when interferon, an "antiviral penicillin," was discovered. Twelve years later, its cancer-inhibiting properties were noted, and its role in cancer treatment has grown over the decades. Nature, not to be outdone, recaptured the lead with Legionnaires' disease, an atypical bacterial pneumonia identified in 1976. It would yield, however, to post-streptomycin antibiotics such as fluoroquinolones, azithromycin, and doxycycline. But then Acquired Immunodeficiency Syndrome (AIDS) erupted on the scene. It was caused by the human immunodeficiency virus (HIV-1) first identified in 1981 and proven to be the cause of AIDS in 1984. AIDS was unresponsive to existing antibiotic and antiviral therapies. Only in 1987, when the FDA released AZT, did AIDS sufferers finally have an effective treatment. In the late 1990s, physicians' off-label use of thalidomide further combatted the "wasting" aspects of the infection.

For the nurses of World War I, the new reality of deadly and untreatable infectious disease belied the promise of late-nineteenth-century bacteriology that, before long, all infectious disease would be eradicated. Now, the nurses and physicians learned, modern bacteriology had profound limits. Medical triumphs, they came to realize, could never be more than partial triumphs linked to the prevention and treatment of specific diseases. The influenza pandemic of 1918 was not among them.

The nurses of World War I were trained and conditioned to nurse on, whatever the odds. The need to remain active was always paramount; activity per se was essential to their personal well-being. We see this again and again in accounts of nurses risking their lives and nursing on during bombing raids that brought the war right to the hospitals. One such account is provided by Helen Boylston, who writes of a combination artillery and air assault on her field hospital in Étaples in May 1918. The assault left patients and nurses alike "frantic with terror," and there appeared at the door of Boylston's ward an off-duty nurse:

> She shivered a little, and smiled at us. "I couldn't stay in my room," she said. "I was so scared, and Gertrude was under the bed, screaming. I couldn't stand it, and I thought if I came over here with the boys, who would need me, I'd be all right."[62]

Several months later, these same nurses, witnessing the death of influenza patients day after day, confronted an enemy no less terrifying. For the severely infected, the nurses' supportive care made no difference; the nurses were stymied, their activity tantamount to inactivity. The worst of it was that the influenza was insidious. It infiltrated the ranks and turned formerly healthy soldiers into conventionally sick soldiers who, at first glance, had developed ordinary respiratory infections. But the infections intensified with lightning speed, and the severely infected quickly became deathly ill and died. There was no mutilation, no dismemberment, no visible internal organs or protruding intestines, no massive facial disfigurement from poison gas. The singularity of the influenza resided partly in its very banality; call it the banality of catastrophe.[63]

The nurses were the advance guard on the nonsurgical frontline, and they absorbed the brunt of the pandemic's fury. It also, inevitably, seeped into the ranks of the nurses, making many of them seriously ill, consigning more still to inactivity, and threatening their collective sense of efficacy and professional self-worth. The nurses' fear of death was real: Their mortality rate was similar to that of American soldiers, which made it 60 percent higher than that of U.S. Army medical officers and four times higher than that of British military nurses.[64] In these several, interrelated ways, pandemic influenza brought the American nurses right into the storm center of medical modernity, at once triumphant and unhappy.

7

Onward

"I can still hear the tramp of stretcher-bearers"[1]

At war's end the American nurses, like their sister soldiers of care in other nations, went their separate ways. Like the soldiers, they were briefly celebrated for service to the nation. Three American nurses, Julia Stimson among them, received the Distinguished Service Cross, the nation's second highest medal for gallantry, while 23 others received the Distinguished Service Medal, the highest decoration awarded to noncombatants.

But decorated or not, the overwhelming majority of nurses returned to civilian lives that may or may not have entailed further nursing. After the war, that is, they ceased functioning as a cohort. The solidarity that had pulled them into forms of nursing practice barely conceivable before the war began to fade, as group identities molded in times of crisis typically do. The American nurses on the Western front, after all, assumed treatment initiatives far in advance of what was expected—or permitted—of nurses. Absent the experiential anchorage provided by wartime exigencies, the nurses fell back into roles consistent with conventional home front understandings of what early-twentieth-century nurses did. These understandings effectively bracketed the kind of nursing called for off the battlefields of Europe as aberrational. Some World War I nurses stayed in the field as redefined by medical and hospital authorities back home. Others left clinical nursing behind and charted new paths in contiguous fields such as public health. Still others left the field but continued to provide nursing care when called on by members of their communities. A few took extended "time outs" from nursing, only

155

to return to it later in life. And some left the workplace for marriage and children; for them the Great War provided more than enough nursing for a lifetime. All of which is to say that the American nurses of the Great War resumed their lives, unmoored from the collective consciousness that for a time propelled them into the realm of what, beginning in the 1970s, was termed advanced practice nursing.

Among the nurses whose wartime experiences enter into the preceding chapters, several segued into full-time civilian nursing positions. At one end of the spectrum, there is Julia Stimson, who ended the war as superintendent of the Army Nursing Corps and became the first Army woman to attain the rank of major. Stimson remained in the Army until 1937, and a year later began a six-year term as president of the American Nursing Association. Following America's entry into the next World War, she became chief of the Nursing Council on National Defense, in which capacity she recruited a new generation of army nurses headed overseas. No less decorated than Stimson was Isabel Anderson, who received the American Red Cross Service Medal, the French Croix de Guerre, and the Medal of Elisabeth of Belgium. Anderson's great wealth never interfered with her social-mindedness. She returned home and immediately volunteered to nurse victims of the raging flu epidemic and then, with her husband, became active in patriotic hereditarian societies such as the Daughters of the American Revolution. At the opposite end of the spectrum, Grace McDougall who, like Stimson and Anderson, earned several medals, had had enough. She moved to Rhodesia with her husband, had three children, farmed the land, and wrote two books. Shirley Millard (née Shirley Eastham), the Red Cross nurse who served in a French field hospital, returned to her native Oregon and married Alfred Millard, Jr. Of her life thereafter there is no record, beyond the fact of her divorce in 1931 and publication of her war memoir *I Saw Them Die* five years later. Helen Fairchild, whose Pennsylvania Hospital Red Cross Unit shared space on the *SS St. Paul* with Julia Stimson's St. Louis unit in the spring of 1917, had a history of abdominal pain that worsened overseas. On January 13, 1919, surgeons operated on her for what x-rays showed to be a large gastric ulcer blocking her pylorus. She died five days later from liver-related complications that followed the use of chloroform to anesthetize her.

Helen Dore Boylston stayed in full-time nursing as head of an outpatient department and instructor of anesthesiology at Massachusetts General Hospital; she later worked as a psychiatric nurse in New York City. Then, following a three-year stint with the Red Cross in Europe from 1921 to1924, she travelled through Europe before settling down in the United States. Between 1936 and 1951, she authored seven "Sue Barton" novels, a popular book series aimed at adolescent girls that followed the trials and tribulations of Nurse Barton through her training and career. Grace Anderson retired from nursing until the late 1930s, when she became a registered nurse in California and with her husband, a former Army surgeon, opened a private emergency hospital. In her later years, she volunteered at a VA Wadsworth Hospital and became active with the League of Women Voters. Alice M. O'Brien, an inveterate traveler for whom postwar trips to Japan and China and later to Africa supplemented regular visits to Europe, became active in a newly formed women's group in her native Minnesota before joining her brother in taking over her father's business in 1925. But her business interests never interfered with advocacy of causes important to her, especially the Children's Hospital of St. Paul, and Camp Courage, a summer camp for children and adults with disabilities. Of Kate Norman Derr, whose *'Mademoiselle Miss'* was published in 1916 without her knowledge by friends in New Brunswick, New Jersey, we know only that she continued to nurse French soldiers and provide aid to indigent French citizens into 1919, at which time she returned to New Brunswick and married Paul Perrot in November of that year.

Among the Canadian nurses, some trained and working in the United States, Laura Holland achieved distinction commensurate with Stimson's, albeit in the civilian sphere. After serving in Lemnos during the Salonika campaign, she left nursing and studied social welfare at Boston's Simmons College. She went on to become Director of Nursing and Emergency Department of the Ontario Division of the Red Cross Society and, then in 1923 Director of the Welfare Division of the Public Health Department of Toronto. She ended her career as the first woman advisor to the Minister of Health and Welfare. Clare Gass returned to Montreal and moved into social work, working in the Social Service Department of Montreal General Hospital for 28 years. Kate Wilson, who contracted influenza late in 1916, returned to Canada in January 1917 and later in the year married Robert Simmie, the Lieutenant (later Captain) she met in France while convalescing. Six children later, at the outbreak of World War II, she became involved with the Red Cross and, following her husband's death in 1948, became a public health nurse in Wiarton, Ontario until retirement.

Alice Isaacson, a naturalized American citizen who nursed in France with the Canadian Army Medical Corps until May 1920, was awarded the Croix de Guerre by the French government. In 1922, after successive short-term jobs with veterans in England and Toronto, she relocated to Ithaca, New York and became the university nurse of Cornell University until her retirement in 1944. Fanny Cluett returned to Newfoundland and resumed teaching in her village of Belleoram, occasionally sharing souvenirs from the war, like her gas mask, with her students. She was in constant demand for private nursing and did her best to accommodate. Ella Mae Bongard returned to Canada, where she married Wilfred Scott in December 1921 and had two sons. She was content to remain at home during World War II, when her husband and both sons served, respectively, in the Canadian Army and Royal Canadian Air Force.

After the war, Nursing Sister Edith Appleton settled in London, where she nursed at Bradford College and cared for her elderly mother. Then in 1923, at the urging of Maud McCarthy, her former chief, she served with Britain's Territorial Force Nursing Service. Kate Luard, a veteran of the Anglo-Boer War and Head Sister at No. 32 CCS during the Battle of Passchendaele, received the Royal Red Cross and Bar (rarely awarded) for her service on the Western front. Having lost her brother Frank during the invasion of Gallipoli in 1915, she left military nursing after the Armistice to care for her ill father, who died in 1919. She nursed on at South London Hospital for Women and then as house matron at a private boys' school before retiring and living with two of her sisters. Dorothea Crewdson was among the nurses who never came home. In the summer of 1918, while serving in Étaples, she suffered severe shrapnel wounds during bombing by German aircraft, but refused treatment in order to care for the patients. She never recovered from her injuries and died of peritonitis the following March. For her gallantry and devotion to duty during the German attack, she posthumously received the Military Medal.

Among the American nurses who stayed in nursing after the war, there is no indication that the profession to which they returned differed from the field they had left several years earlier. There is no evidence, that is, that their nursing activities on the Western front had any impact on the nature of their profession back home. Certainly, they were not heralded as ushering in a new era of nursing practice. American nursing continued on its slow evolutionary course right into the 1960s, when advanced nursing practice finally left the hospital setting and became office-based, especially in the realm of primary care. This development marked the birth of the nurse practitioner movement, which began with the pediatric nurse practitioner training program at the University of Colorado in the mid–1960s and, over the next two decades, empowered American nursing to free itself from what many nurses saw as the profession's bondage to organized medicine, with its long-held belief in the subordinate role of nurses as "physician extenders."[2]

It was the Vietnam War that provided impetus to this new trajectory. But things were far different after the Great War. In 1919, when most American nurses returned home, there was only a fledgling American Nurses Association, founded as the Nurses Associated Alumnae in 1898 and renamed in 1911. American nurses' subservience to physicians was codified in a version of the Nightingale pledge written in 1893 and recited when nurses were pinned at their graduation.[3] Self-evidently the ANA of postwar America was not exactly a wellspring of support for individual nurse initiative; indeed, it admitted only state societies, not individuals—this a strategy for excluding trained African American nurses who were excluded from their state societies. So there was no institutional support for an expansion of nursing practice, even if returning military nurses had been of a mind to seek it.[4] During the 1920s American hospitals may have been appreciative of what returning military nurses had endured and the qualities of character the war had elicited. But that is where matters ended. There is no evidence physicians, hospital administrators, or senior staff nurses were interested in the diagnostic and procedural skills the nurses had acquired in Europe or in how these skills could be employed in American hospitals.

Combat nursing, for self-evident reasons, has always been ahead of the curve. The rigors and hardships of service abroad are compensated not only by the rank and respect accorded nurses, but by treatment prerogatives commensurate with their training and skill. The World War I nurses were not the only combat nurses to resume civilian nursing roles back in American hospitals. Back in the States after returning home from service in the Burma-China-India theater during World War II, LaVonne Camp took a position as staff nurse in a community hospital in Glen Ridge, New Jersey. On her first day, the head nurse, who did not believe Camp could read charts and understand diagnoses, had her clean windows and beds. "It became clear," she later wrote, "that my professional colleagues who had remained in civilian positions had little appreciation for the liberating effect the war had on those of us who served our country."[5]

If we jump forward a half century from World War I to America's war in Vietnam, we see a similar unwillingness on the part of hospitals to bend much less change their rules to accommodate nurses' combat experience. Vietnam nurses returning to the States were both bemused and miffed when their new hospitals refused to let them start IVs (intravenous therapy via venous puncture) until they had taken the hospital's own IV training class. "While in Vietnam," remarked one such nurse, "we often had to start IVs on our knees holding a flashlight in the dark!"[6] More serious violations of hospital protocol could get returning nurses in trouble. Their wartime experience had made inserting chest tubes and performing tracheotomies routine. Back in the States, however, such initiatives exceeded the scope of nursing practice. Military nurses' training and experience overseas had nothing to do with it. It was as if they were expected to forget all they had learned.[7] Other nurses, for whom the Vietnam experience left open wounds—PTSD symptoms, anger, anxiety, an unresolvable sense of betrayal by the military and the public—could not negotiate the gulf between military and civilian practice. For Bernadette Harrod, hard-won surgical skills were among the casualties of a war whose traumatizing impact continued back home. Absent military recognition, any expression of public appreciation, or a support network of female Vietnam vets, Harrod was among those who went "undercover" in an ill-fated effort to get her war experience behind her. Her surgical skills went undercover with her:

> I had developed skills in the OR that I could never use stateside. I could clamp and cut and suture. The deep sense of equality that I knew on the OR team was gone forever. I couldn't go through the double doors to surgery anymore and be a second-class citizen, a handmaiden, a passer of instruments. So I did what many others did, despite the skills that they had painfully acquired in Vietnam: I denied my own experience, and I never went into the OR again.[8]

This story ends with the nurses of Vietnam, but the expanded scope of practice of military nurses serving in American wars does not. Army nurses serving in Iraq and Afghanistan mention insertion of chest tubes, endotracheal intubation, and tracheotomies among the surgical procedures relegated to them overseas. "When you have only two surgeons and have 15 critical patients," remarked an army nurse who served in Iraq, "you end up doing more than the nurses do in a stateside ICU or trauma unit." "Civilian wise," another added for emphasis, such procedures were not part of a nurse's job description. Other surgical activities assigned to nurses in emergency areas and deemed worthy of mention—debriding wounds, exploring wounds and removing shrapnel, suturing wounds—are the same activities undertaken by nurses in reception huts on the Western front a century earlier.[9]

• • •

The progress of American nursing in the 1920s was limited to the organizational and educational fronts. In 1923, the first four free-standing baccalaureate programs in nursing were established. Three years later, the Committee on Grading of the National League of Nursing Educators began an eight-year survey that identified over-production of graduates as the root cause of the profession's problems. Its final report of 1934 recommended, inter alia, reduction in the number of nursing schools, higher entrance requirements, and the separation of nursing education and nursing services in hospitals.[10] The Commission's recommendations, of course, were responsive to the Great Depression, when over 800 hospitals closed their schools of nursing and gave private duty nurses temporary staff positions to perform the work previously allocated to student nurses.[11] Faced with drastically reduced job opportunities, graduate nurses who wanted to work at all were often forced to take low-paying jobs as floor nurses or enter the private duty sector.

So both administrative and economic forces were aligned against the veterans of the Western front, whatever their array of treatment skills. The organization of nurse anesthetists after the war is the major exception to this claim. This was not the case in Britain, where nurse anesthetists of the Western front, some trained by Americans, were kept out of operating rooms back home. Only physicians administered general anesthesia in postwar Britain. But in America things went forward. In 1923, at the instigation of Agatha Hodgins, graduates of the Lakeside School of Anesthesia formed an Alumnae Association. In 1926, the group reorganized and Hodgins proposed a plan for a national organization of nurse anesthetists. But it was only in June 1931, with the nation now gripped by the Depression, that the American Association of Nurse Anesthetists held its first organizational meeting. Even this counterexample is misleading, however, since the nurses' role as pioneer anesthetists with the training and skill to employ the new generation of gas anesthesia machines was well established before the Great War. Further, the Association was reactive to the Depression-era maneuvering of physician anesthetists, now intent on securing their income by eliminating nurse competition. The nurse anesthetists came together to safeguard their prerogative to practice as anesthetists, to establish their own educational and accreditation standards, thereby preventing absorption into the American Nursing Association as a mere "section."[12]

• • •

Back home America's Great War nurses received their fair share of accolades in the form of military decorations, professional awards, and public and private celebrations. For all concerned, they were courageous exemplars of the Nightingalean creed. They nursed on under circumstances that ranged from difficult to dire, often risking life and limb while caring for their patients. But the special competencies achieved by these nurses, which went well beyond the general skills imparted by three years of hospital training, were less well understood, least of all by the public that welcomed them back to traditional female roles, nursing and otherwise.

What acknowledgment they received for service beyond the pale of traditional nursing came from Congress and the Army. In 1920, scarcely a year after the Paris Peace Treaty, Congress passed the Army Reorganization Act. In tribute to the performance of Army nurses in the war, the Act granted them "relative rank," which made them commissioned officers, albeit officers of a lesser order without the pay or benefits of real (i.e., male) officers. The Act also permitted them to receive specialized training in fields such as anesthesia at civilian hospitals while remaining on Army payrolls. The nurses of World War I had acquired procedural competence on the job. Stateside specialty training meant that many Army nurses in the next world war would arrive in battle zones with an array of procedural skills in hand.

When America entered the Second World War two decades later, the Army followed suit by sending medical and nursing corps inductees alike to four-week training courses at centers throughout the country. Here nurses attended lectures on triaging, another skill their Great War predecessors had learned from other nurses in the reception huts of casualty clearing stations and field hospitals. During World War II nursing skills were less an issue than the nurses' readiness for life in a combat zone. Four weeks of preliminary training, two of which were spent on wards, were not found sufficient to transform civilian nurses into Army nurses. So beginning in late 1943 the Training Division, Office of the Surgeon General instituted a "Battle School for Nurses" in Shrivenham, England. American nurses completed its program before being assigned to their hospital units.[13]

• • •

Issues of gender and sexuality have figured only peripherally in this study of nursing practice, the single exception concerning the nurse's hand as an instrument of caregiving.[14] But consideration of female touch is merely one aspect of the various ways in which gender enters into nursing. Self-evidently, World War I nursing was a gendered affair. The professionalization of nursing that followed the Civil War was grafted onto a gendered understanding of what nursing was. Beginning with the first hospital training programs of 1873, nursing became a profession, but as a profession, it was little more than the scientific fine-tuning of women's domestic work. This was the lesson that Florence Nightingale brought back from the Crimea and codified in her *Notes on Nursing: What It Is and What It Is Not* (1859). For Nightingale, what would become professional nursing was simply "true nursing" or "sanitary nursing," by which she meant the womanly provision of comfort care enlarged by sanitary science and scientifically informed bedside observation. Treat patients like good mothers treat their sick children, she adjured, keeping them warm, dry, and well nourished. And before all else, spare them the foul air of sealed rooms, the underlying culprit in many a child's prolonged illness and death. Open the windows, bring in fresh outside air, and the body will do the rest.[15] This was all woman's work, pure and simple. Indeed, the professionalization of nursing after the Civil War was authorized *by men* appreciative of the usefulness of such domestic precepts in the hospitals of the North. Wounded and dying soldiers, Union officers and surgeons found, eagerly sought and benefited from the ministrations of nurses who were surrogate mothers, wives, and sisters.

A generation later, when Isabel Hampton Robb published her influential textbooks on nursing practice and nursing ethics, respectively, comfort care had been enlarged by the growth of scientific medicine, especially bacteriology, during the final decade of the nineteenth century. But the gendered assumptions of mid-century pioneers such as Nightingale and Clara Barton were left untouched. Nursing care, as Robb understood it, was still woman's work, the difference being that by the 1890s the rigorous demands of hospital care meant that nurse training schools sought "a higher order of woman to meet these requirements." Only by enrolling young women of the highest standards in nursing schools, she opined, would the institutions and communities in which trained nurses toiled "show forth the influence of that 'sweet ordering, arrangement and decision' that are woman's chief prerogatives."[16]

Despite the concerted effort of Alice McGee to sever the connection between nursing and Nightingalean assumptions during and after the Spanish-American War, the "domestic sphere" rationale of nursing remained in force at the time of the Great War. The expansion of nursing activity into new realms of clinical decision-making and technology-driven intervention was simply added to the belief that nurses were womanly providers. The nurses whose hands administered gas anesthesia, assisted in major surgery, performed minor bedside surgery, and monitored the Dakin-Carrel apparatus were the same nurses whose womanly touch was a vital instrument of caring.

The American nurses of the Great War, competent in ways unimaginable to the founders of nurse training programs, were simply New Nightingales, their identity as scientifically trained providers grafted onto timeworn Nightingalean assumptions about the gentle art of womanly healing. This is because the Nightingalean assumptions had less to do with discrete nursing practices than with a set of values that guided nurses into nursing and from there in the direction of listening, understanding, withholding judgment, and comforting—what we now gather into the notion of patient-centered care. These values continued to guide nursing activity through the Great War—whether the activity was simple comfort care at the bedside or more recent medicalized additions to the nurse's armamentarium. All such activities, patients discovered, could be aligned with a woman's caring touch.

◆ ◆ ◆

This integration of scientific nursing and Nightingalean values remained powerful in World War II. To be sure, the values shifted somewhat, as a new, youthful cohort of military nurses, unburdened by the beatific mythology of European Sisters, nursed wounded soldiers in the more prosaic role of sisters and wives, girlfriends and gals. But the shift left the Nightingalean premise largely intact. A 1944 U.S. Army nurse recruiting film drove the premise home: "Professionally skilled and capable," intones the narrator, "in her [the Army nurse] there is the tenderness of all women, of mother and sister and friend. Her voice and touch lend encouragement, instill hope. It's the surgeon who saves a man's life; it's the nurse whose tender care helps him to live."[17]

One need not search far to find instances of American nurses of World War II "mothering" their youthful male patients, but the mothering seems, on the whole, more attenuated than that of the Great War nurses. The American nurses of World War II entered service as part of an Army Nursing Corps that, in relation to that of 1917, was highly organized, well structured, and ceded by all to be an essential component of the American military. Individual nurses were women of faith, certainly, but the religious moorings of nursing practice were greatly loosened and for many, perhaps, nonexistent. In their place, there was the mature professionalism that came into existence during the interwar years.

Nurse specialization went hand in hand with the heightened technological component of nursing in general. World War I nurses' responsibility for mixing Dakin's solution and titrating its flow through Carrel's complicated apparatus of valves and tubes was prescient of the technological transformation of combat nursing in World War II, when routine bedside care went beyond sponge baths, medication, morphine injections, wound dressings, and comforting talk. It now included transfusions of plasma and whole blood, drawing blood and ordering laboratory studies, and charting the results that came back. Blood transfusions, we have noted, were performed in the final years of World War I, but only by physicians in base and general hospitals off the front. But other forms of intravenous (IV) or "drip" therapy—the injection of bodily fluids or medications directly into veins—only became practical in the 1930s, after Columbia University researchers Samuel Hirshfeld, Harold Hyman, and Justine Wanger demonstrated the relationship of the speed of infusion to the success of IV therapy.[18] In World War II, nurses usually assisted physicians in starting IVs though, when circumstances required, they were capable of performing the venous needle insertions and beginning IV drips by themselves "Can you give IV?" a physician asked Julia Polchlopek Scott, an Army nurse receiving wounded on Saipan during the battle for Iwo Jima in the summer of 1944. "I thought he was crazy," she answered, "because none of the nurses had. He gave me five minutes of instruction so he could go on with other things, and I learned to do intravenous anesthesia on-the-job. It was scary. I stopped breathing with every one of them, then took a deep breath when they did."[19]

•   •   •

In the Second World War, nurses' self-confidence, teamed with a resolutely patient-centered orientation, could bring them to open conflict with physicians. Sally Hitchcock, serving on the Philippine island of Leyte in early 1945, wrote home of an instance when the physician who was her ward officer was so dismissive of a patient's severe lower-right abdominal pain that he refused to order appropriate lab studies and would not even examine the young man. Hitchcock took matters into her own hands and ordered emergency blood work that revealed a drastically elevated white cell count. The soldier was rushed to surgery where, she wrote home, "a red-hot appendix was removed." The ward officer was livid, but for questioning her ward officer's judgment and proceeding on her own, Hitchcock was commended and received a promotion. Six months later, she confronted another ward physician who refused to do anything for an acute patient for two consecutive nights. When she continued to "raise the roof" the following day, action followed: The patient was operated on for intestinal blockage.[20] Aloha Sanchez, an Army Air Force nurse based in China, informed doctors that her hospital was running out of oxygen three days before the supply would be exhausted. When oxygen failed to arrive and an American soldier died on account of it, she and her partner "had had it, and we complained at the top," getting transferred to the base for their efforts.[21] It is difficult to envision such instances of confrontations in the Great War.

In World War II the rushes of the Great War gave way to large-scale, often amphibious invasions in the various theaters of war. Following the Japanese attack on Pearl Harbor and landing on the Philippines island of Luzon 17 days later, American nurses, in scenes reminiscent of the Great War, confronted overwhelming numbers of casualties brought to hospital doors. Nurses coped with the crisis by distributing emergency procedures in the manner of an assembly line. In language that could be applied equally to Flanders in 1917, a nurse at Schofield Barracks Hospital on Oahu recalled the scene just days after the Japanese attack: "the stream of casualties was so overwhelming that they could not separate the living from the dead, bodies were piling up like cordwood wherever there was space." Nurses, doctors, and medics alike were especially appalled by "the many wounded men who were missing arms and legs, and those so seriously burned 'the medical staff was amazed they were still alive when they were brought in.'" And in an aside that evokes the bloodbath through which the Great War nurses occasionally waded, she adds that "blood seemed to work its way into every nook and cranny of the hospital."[22]

In the aftermath of Pearl Harbor, American nurses and doctors often worked out of temporary hospitals set up in schools or primitive wooden buildings. One nurse would fill syringes with morphine sulphate, stimulants, and tetanus vaccine while another went from bed to bed giving the injections; a third nurse hung intravenous fluids and blood transfusions from nails in the rafters. Depending on the hospital and the availability of supplies, a fourth nurse could be tasked with going from bed to bed, doing a preliminary assessment and cleaning open wounds, into which sulfanilamide power was directly applied before the wounds were covered with a heavy gauze dressing.[23] D-Day, the allied invasion of Europe from the beachheads of Normandy beginning June 6, 1944, was another gigantic reprise of the World War I rushes. At the 91st field hospital, which began receiving casualties five days later, 251 patients were admitted in the first 13 hours and 2,142 patients over the next 17 days. As surgeons operated around the clock, nurses and the technicians they supervised transfused plasma and whole blood in addition to giving pain medication.[24]

During the later stages of the war in the Pacific, the allied retaking of islands in the southwest Pacific occupied by Japan since 1941, nurses stepped into the breach yet again, reminding us of the manner in which their Great War predecessors likewise rose to the occasion after the epic battles of the Somme and the Marne. Sally Hitchcock, working out of the 61st General Hospital in Hollandia, New Guinea, recalled the situation that befell nurses following MacArthur's invasion of Leyte, in the Philippines, in October 1944. The intense fighting meant that rotating teams of hospital doctors and nurses had been moved north to help cope with the wounded flowing into field hospitals. This left the general hospitals drastically short-handed and meant: "We have to do what they [the doctors] had been doing. Every day I thank God for all the training I received, my operating room months, my surgery and all the theory I have had, because I was asked to do things I've never done and there is no one else to do them."[25] Several weeks later, with the medical staff still depleted, she was more explicit about the things she was now called on to do: "I never thought I'd be able to probe and dig and scrub open wounds. You have to do it. In one draining wound, I probed and pulled out a piece of shrapnel." And then, speaking of one of her "special patients," she elaborated in still greater detail on her bedside doctoring:

> He has a wound that goes diagonally all the way through his thigh. We have to probe it from both sides to keep it open to heal from the inside out. When there is no longer a doctor to do this, I have to do it. The shrapnel sticking out of his leg caught on the sheets so I was told to remove the pieces, to do the best I could. There were no doctors available at this time. I washed the areas, made a nick with a scalpel, and removed the slivers. Washing carefully with azochloromide, I fired some butterflies and closed the wounds. They are healing well. I am pleased.[26]

Such beside surgical care, we have seen, was not uncommon three decades earlier on the Western front, where surgeons were far fewer and minor surgical tasks were routinely relegated to nurses. European Sisters and American nurses wielded scalpels then too, and with considerable skill. It is in the realm of drug therapy that World War II represented a quantum leap beyond World War I, and nursing care was greatly influenced by it. For the nurses of World War II had sulfa drugs, the first modern antibiotics, and Atabrine, an effective malarial preventive. Beginning in 1943, moreover, they had penicillin, a game changer, a broad spectrum antibiotic effective in treating wound infections and infectious diseases alike. Equally effective in treating pneumonia and venereal disease, penicillin also saved thousands of GIs from the gas gangrene that plagued the Doughboys and was the bane of their nurses.

In mid–1945 Sally Hitchcock, still nursing in a field hospital in Leyte, recalled an instance when a penicillin shortage threated reamputation for a soldier with a gangrenous leg. The infection had already claimed his lower leg, and surgeons and nurses were now desperate to avoid removing his thigh. To provide the necessary doses for the patient, they not only reduced penicillin doses for all other patients, first on the ward and then in the hospital, but combed other hospitals on the island for additional supplies. With the regular penicillin injections that resulted from these initiatives, the soldier's infection was contained, saving his thigh and probably his life.[27] Such instances render tangible the notion of a miracle drug. With penicillin in hand, hot poultices and sponge baths to relieve fever became things of the past; the very notion of "good old-fashioned nursing" had, for some, become superfluous.[28] Similarly, the ingenious ways in which World War I surgeons and nurses irrigated infected wounds with an assortment of antiseptics, such as Dakin's solution, were consigned to the dustbin of medical history.

Sulfa drugs and Atabrine, ironically, were gifts of the German dye industry. The former came from the I. G. Farben Division of what was then the Bayer Dye Works. Bayer had the financial resources and foresight to support the research of Gerhardt Domagk, whose unswerving commitment to finding an effective anti-microbial agent led to his discovery in 1932 of a dye (initially identified as KI-695, then as Kl730) capable of destroying the streptococcal bacteria that caused infections ranging from sore throats to puerperal sepsis (childbed fever) to blood poisoning to erysipelas, a deep skin infection. The dye also proved effective with meningitis and pneumonia. The first sulfa drug, Prontosil, was released in Germany in 1935, the same year that French researchers at the Pasteur Institute determined that sulfapyridine, a small molecule that was part of the dye compound, was responsible for its anti-microbial properties. It was released in the U.S. in 1936 and widely used throughout World War II, when every American soldier received a first-aid kit with both sulfa pills and sulfa powder; they were instructed to sprinkle the powder on any open wound. Penicillin, which became available only in mid–1943, in time for D-Day, was a far more effective drug with a far broader spectrum of activity than the sulfa drugs; for nurses and doctors, not to mention untold patients, it was a godsend.

Quinacrine (trade name Atabrine), a synthetic antimalarial also developed at Bayer in 1931, was an effective substitute for quinine, which, following the German occupation of Holland and Japanese occupation of the quinine-producing areas of Southeast Asia, was no longer available to America. Like sulfa pills, Atabrine was liberally dispensed on the wards to prevent malaria. Nurses began taking it on the transport ships; indeed, the Atabrine on the breakfast table was an unmistakable sign of where they were heading.[29] But American soldiers initially resisted taking the drug. They disliked its yellowing effect on their skin and, heeding Japanese propaganda, feared it would leave them sterile. Hospitalized GIs, intent on extending their hospital stays, were known to spit out Atabrine pills. Even nurses occasionally refused to take the daily pill, especially after their yellow skin darkened into a deep and, they believed, unattractive tan. And nurses, no less than soldiers, contracted malaria as a result. Lavonne Camp, a veteran of the China-Burma-India campaign stationed in Ledo, India, recalled that nurses who failed to take their morning pill could be court martialed.[30] After anti-malarial researchers at New York's Goldwater Memorial Hospital, led by James Shannon, arrived at a new dosage schedule by determining how to measure Atabrine levels in the blood, resistance lessened and the drug came to the aid of thousands of Americans abroad.

Taken together sulfa drugs, Atabrine, and penicillin dramatically eased the palliative burden on combat nurses caring for soldiers with serious infections, both wound-related and systemic. Prevention became integral to their modus operandi, on and off the wards. Soldiers and nurses alike were given Atabrine pills on the transport ships that carried them to Europe.[31] Once in their hospitals, nurses became part of the new drug culture, dispensing sulfa pills with ease throughout the day. Every soldier on the base received two sulfa pills every morning, recalled one.[32] The demands on nurses caring for malaria patients in the pre–Atabrine era is captured, with no small irony, by a World War II nurse. Here is Sally Hitchcock, reporting on her work on an isolation ward during her training course at Fort Devens in Ayer, Massachusetts. She is writing, one surmises, of a soldier who either had not been given, or not taken, Atabrine preventively. "So many guys on this floor were sent home with malaria," she wrote her parents. "They are so sick when the chills hit and we have to give ice water sponges, have a fan blowing on them trying to get the spiking temperatures down. The fevers are so high! It is a brand new experience." Hitchcock herself, along with all the other nurses and medical officers, took an Atabrine pill every morning at breakfast before going to work.[33]

Atabrine was effective, but in the wards of field and general hospitals the term "miraculous" was reserved for the new antibiotics. Even under the most dire circumstances, such as the primitive Malinta Tunnel Hospital on Corregidor Island, adequate care could be provided owing to sufficient supplies of sulfa drugs.[34] Beginning in 1943, administering penicillin injections every three or four hours became as time-consuming as turning on and off the valves of the Carrel apparatus at bedside had been for the Great War nurses. "It would take hours," recalled a veteran nurse of both the North African and Italian campaigns. "You would finish one round of penicillin and it would be time to start another dose." She recalled giving intramuscular injections on a three-hour schedule, with the medic running back and forth to sterilize the needles. To make the process even more time-consuming still, nurses had to prepare injectable penicillin solution from the powder they were shipped.[35] For a raft of systemic infections, on the other hand, where antiseptic drainage was not a possibility, World War I nurses had little more to offer than palliation, keeping patients warm, dry, and hydrated, and bringing down their fevers with ice and sponge baths.

Following an experimental flight carrying wounded soldiers from Karachi, India to the United States in January 1943,[36] Army Air Force instructors at Bowman Air Field in Louisville, Kentucky began training Army nurses to accompany casualties on medical evacuation flights in the South Pacific. The flights took the wounded from New Guinea to air bases in Australia or from Burma to India. At first, absent dedicated hospital planes, the nurses and medical techs were crammed into cargo planes and let off one or two at a time whenever the plane landed. In short order, however, dedicated C-47 Douglas Skytrains were used for medical evacuation. Despite being unmarked, the planes were at considerable risk of Japanese attack. With no physicians on board, the plane's single flight nurse assumed full responsibility for treating up to 54 seriously wounded GIs. In the course of such flights, nurses had to cope with GIs who went into shock or developed signs of hemorrhage. To provide for nonmedical contingencies, moreover, flight nurses carried .45 caliber pistols they were trained to use.[37] Beginning in June 1944, Medical Air Evacuation Squadrons based in England proved their worth by evacuating severe battle casualties from the Normandy invasion to hospitals in England and then, beginning in November, across the Atlantic to the United States. Over the summer months alone, more than 20,000 patients were evacuated from France by air.[38] By the time of the Korean War, America's air evacuation service incorporated helicopters, initially light craft able to evacuate only 1–2 wounded soldiers, and then in Vietnam, more substantial Huey helicopters that carried 6–9 wounded at a time to hospitals.

The reliance of air evacuation on flight nurses signals a domain of medical responsibility outside the realm of World War I nurses. The role of nurses on the hospital trains of the First World War, enormous affairs of up to 16 cars that carry up to 500 injured and sick troops from aid stations to base hospitals, provides the weakest of analogies. The Army medical department, following the British example, assigned only three medical officers and three nurses (later changed to two medical officers and four nurses) to each train. What meager care the wounded received came from 30 or so ward car orderlies, whose briefing came from the train commander during his inspection right after departure. How much could he convey to the enlisted men about the special needs of individual soldiers among the hundreds being evacuated? At stops along the way, military doctors wait for trains to arrive, removing the desperately ill, "those whom a few miles more would finish forever." At larger stations, tents are set up right off the platform—one for operations that cannot wait, one for dressings, one for food, one for the dying, and one for the dead. Unsurprisingly, the train commander's report to his superiors always notes the number of entrained soldiers who should never have left the front and those who died before reaching their destination.[39]

This was not the case with the greatly improved hospital trains of World War II, which often included a train car set aside for surgery and another for wound dressings. And it was certainly not the case for soldiers evacuated to hospitals on C-47 Skytrains. There appears little of Florence Nightingale in the medical authority nurses were assigned in managing their cargo of seriously wounded, all of whom were expected to survive their flights, whatever emergencies might arise over mountains or oceans. And yet, tellingly, the historian Barbara Tomblin titles her interview-based study of Army Nurses Corps in World War II, from which the foregoing summary of flight nursing is drawn, *G.I. Nightingales.*

• • •

America's war in Vietnam is a half century removed from the Great War, a half century of staggering medical and surgical advance. It is surprising, therefore, that in key respects Vietnam nursing was a continuation of the experience of Great War nurses. To be sure, the half century witnessed major achievements. By Vietnam, gender-free professionalisms had taken root. Or so it seemed. America's Vietnam nurses were now commissioned officers with full rank, pay, and benefits. As health care professionals, moreover, they were not only trained to employ advanced technologies that emerged after World War II, but expected to pass on these skills to the medical corpsmen whom they supervised. Indeed, nurse training in the military now entailed the training of corpsmen as a major component.

Separated by a half century and occurring in dramatically different environments, the two wars still provide striking convergences in nurses' modus operandi. Little that occurred in Vietnam was not rehearsed in the casualty clearing stations and field hospitals of the Western front. The "rushes" that followed major offensives on the Front became the "mass casualty situations" of enemy offensives, when soldiers arrived at field hospitals "until litters holding soldiers covered the floor."[40] In Vietnam as in Flanders, nurses were called on to work continuously for two, even three days. Triaging followed the military philosophy worked out in the reception huts of France and Belgium, with nurses again making critical decisions about the order of surgery based on the military objective of "salvaging" as many wounded bodies as possible.

Vietnam nurses were again tasked with deciding which soldiers were beyond saving. The mortuary tents of the Great War became the screened off corners of receiving wards or intensive care units where the dying died. Indeed, the emotional burden on the Vietnam nurses may have been greater still, since they were required to monitor the vital signs of dying soldiers until heart beats ceased.[41] This was skilled nursing, abetted by technology, in the service of death. Unable to undertake treatment or provide pain relief for these soldiers, Vietnam nurses, like their World War I forebears, fell back on the most basic instruments at their disposal—their hands and their voices:

> All a nurse could do was to touch and speak to these men. While listening for a heart-beat, a nurse would hold a man's hands and whisper into his ear. In Vietnam, and in other wars, women learned that nursing was more than healing. The women learned to measure death and soothe the way.[42]

Among soldiers who recovered, nurses faced a burden with which the World War I nurses were intimately acquainted. In Vietnam no less than on the Western front, nurses had to bow to military directives to keep troop levels up. In both wars, nurses struggled with the obligation to send the adequately if precariously healed back to trenches or combat units, respectively. They did so in the knowledge that some would return to them newly wounded, perhaps grievously, while others would die in the field.[43]

Vietnam nurses recorded their conflicts over providing nursing care to wounded enemy combatants and civilians. But American nurses on the Western front experienced the same conflicts in caring for wounded Germans. Nor were the Vietnam nurses the first who, after several months of service, came to humanize the enemy as fellow human sufferers, frightened, helpless, and in need of care. But this was no less true of World War I nurses who cared for German prisoners of war. The ethical obligation was harder in Vietnam. Nurses on the Western front quickly found that German prisoners, with few exceptions, exuded gratitude: "they wouldn't think of running away, haven't had it so good in a long time in spite of some of the awful injuries," remarked Maude Essig in October 1918. Beatrice Hopkinson concurred that German prisoners mostly preferred being British prisoners to fighting: "They said the food and clothing we gave them were much better than they had received in the German Army and cigarettes were almost a thing of the past." And from Base Hospital 15, part of the Hospital Center in Vichy, Elizabeth Lewis wrote home of taking care of, and talking to, appreciative German prisoners.[44]

A half century later, care of prisoners was more challenging. Nurses in Vietnam had to cope with POWs who spoke no English and were unfamiliar with Western nursing practices. Often, they resisted treatment, convinced the American nurses were trying to kill them. The challenge of caring for them was more akin to that of American

World War II nurses in the Pacific who, in the intense fighting to retake north Burma in 1944, could become "squeezed dry of compassion" for the wounded and sick Chinese fighting alongside allied troops. The medical officers at her hospital, recounted LaVonne Telshaw Camp, were even worse: "Theirs was a malignant apathy toward the Chinese patients, for they saw in these men a callous attitude toward human life, and they felt that their compassion was wasted."[45]

At the time of Vietnam, the U.S. Army, despite the equality of rank and pay accorded female officers, had not yet resolved an ongoing crisis of ambivalence about female officers in combat zones. It urgently needed professional nurses and valued them highly. But it continued to wrestle with the biological difference of the sexes, ricocheting between gender-based protectiveness and gender-free indifference. Women soldiers, regardless of rank, remained women in need of male protection, whether or not they sought it. Nurses had to be accompanied by armed escorts whenever they went off base.[46] A report of alleged rape could mean that all American women, officers and enlisted alike, had to have Marine escorts when they walked around their own hospital compound.[47]

Nurse accounts of the time suggest that Army protectiveness had as much to do with the nurses' male comrades as with enemy troops. Women's liberation only went so far in what remained an army of young men, and sexually deprived young men at that. When a red alert signaled an enemy attack, usually at night, male troops rushed to their bunkers. But, at some bases, alert orders for women were changed. Rather than have nurses clad only in pajamas and nightgowns join male comrades in the bunkers, the nurses' Quonset huts were sandbagged to chest height so that they could remain in them during the alerts. The Army's concern, recalled one nurse, "was not that the enemy would 'get us,' but that American soldiers would see us."[48]

The nurses were sexual distractions; the nurses were professional caregivers whose skills were invaluable. The two-sidedness is a hallmark of the American army, and was certainly in evidence throughout the war in Vietnam. The army's protectiveness might have carried greater weight if it were complemented by planning responsive to the biological difference of the sexes. Throughout the war, for example, Army exchanges (PX stores) did not stock feminine hygiene supplies; nurses along with other military women had to have tampons sent from home. A Vietnam nurse interviewed by Elizabeth Norman mused why an entire hospital had only one women's bathroom.[49]

• • •

In their efforts to enter the male world of American medicine in the mid-nineteenth century, pioneer women physicians adopted two opposing strategies of assimilation. On the one hand, we have the touch-comfort-sympathy approach of Elizabeth Blackwell. She assigned women their own feminized domain of medical practice—child care, nonsurgical obstetrics and gynecology, womanly counseling on matters of sanitation, hygiene, and prevention—and advised them to abjure surgery. At the other pole there is the research-oriented, scientific approach of Mary Putnam Jacobi and Marie Zakrezewska, which held that women physicians must be physicians in any and all respects. Only with state-of-the-art training in the medical science (e.g., bacteriology) and treatments (e.g., ovariotomy) of the day, would women docs achieve what they deserved: full parity with medical men. The binary of female physicians as extenders of women's "natural sphere" versus female physicians as physicians pure and simple runs through the second half of the nineteenth century.[50]

At first glance, the American nurses of World War I carried nursing activity into the modern era through the path charted out by Elizabeth Blackwell and her colleagues. That is, they used their womanhood as an asset in the nursing sphere; their maternalism, their touch, their comfort care, their counsel, their ability to calm severely wounded soldiers—all were heightened by the womanly virtues they brought to the reception huts and carried with them in the wards. This understanding of nursing as an extension of women's domestic sphere carries over from the Civil War. The nurse's terms of endearment were unchanged in the Spanish-American War, when American graduate nurses served the military in training camps in the American South and in hospitals, in Cuba and in the Philippines. In his commentary on the medical aspects of the war, we recall, Nicholas Seen lauded the nurses in pure Nightingalean fashion, even to the point of parroting Nightingale: "She [woman] is a born nurse ... endowed with all the qualification, mentally and physically, to take care of the sick."[51]

The Nightingalean vision was alive and well during the Great War. It underlay the Army's acceptance of nurses' crucial role all along the Western front, especially their presence in the casualty clearing stations just a few miles off the front. The curious thing is that the gendered virtues that gave them access to battlefield casualties did not limit them to a feminine sphere of action. Perforce the nurses had unrestricted access to the male bodies brought to them. Gendered nursing aptitude, that is, was not constraining as it had been for all but a few Civil War nurses. The male bodies brought to the comforting hands of female nurses were not simply the bodies of men wracked with typhoid, typhus, malaria, dysentery, diphtheria, influenza, et al. They were bodies that lacked the wholeness of bodies—bodies mutilated, ripped open, missing limbs or faces or chunks of torso, bodies burned up and grossly disfigured from poison gas. The nurses did not use gender as a cloak to shield them from their obligation to nurse decimated male bodies. Rather, they brusquely waved off whatever sensibilities military authorities imputed to their prewar selves. They joined the surgeons and orderlies in doing all they could with the resources of their time and place.

And what exactly did these resources make possible? By the time of the Great War, medical science had hitched its star to laboratory medicine, which is to say, to bacteriology and bacteriological theories of disease transmission. In so doing, it pulled professional nursing into a new epistemological orbit. Great War nurses remained women, blessed with the caring touch of women, but the war taught them—and all the men around them—that female touch placed no limitation on what trained female hands could do, *operationally* speaking. In this sense, the nurses of the Great War inherited the mantle of Mary Putnam Jacobi and Marie Zakrezewska, for whom the treatment prerogatives of women physicians had to be coextensive with those of male colleagues. The proceduralism of which we have written was neither constrained nor enhanced by gender. Rather, it was coordinate with what was expected of scientifically trained caregivers in the second decade of the twentieth century. That the nurses nursed on as scientifically as they could under conditions of privation, discomfort, and illness; that they waded through pools of blood and ponds of mud; that they risked their lives during enemy shellings; that they worked through their own bouts of depression and shell shock—these things should have surprised everyone but should have surprised no one.

• • •

At the remove of a century, with several waves of feminism under our societal belt and nursing in combat zones a longstanding fact of military life, it is difficult to grasp the magnitude of what the World War I nurses accomplished. They not only stepped into their historical moment but, in so doing, jumped from one professional orbit to another, aligning with the notion of professional nursing a range of medical, surgical, and psychotherapeutic interventions formerly reserved for physicians. Many of the nurses were lightly trained volunteers, and even the graduate nurses who had completed their three-year training programs assumed responsibilities far beyond anything their instructors prepared them for. In so doing, they broke through, however fleetingly and far from home, the gendered constraints of an era scarcely free of Victorian sensibilities about single young women and the things they could and could not do, especially with regard to the male body. When an artillery shell landed in the midst of a group of men gathered outside a tunnel entrance, nurses were at the ready. What followed were

> hours of giving injections, anesthetizing, ripping off clothes, stitching gaping wounds, of amputations, sterilizing instruments, settling the treated patients in their beds, covering the wounded we could not save. I had still not grown accustomed to seeing people torn and bleeding and dying in numbers like these.[52]

But wait. This is not a nurse on the Western front in 1917. It is Juanita Redmond, an American army nurse on the island of Corregidor in the Philippines, and she is reporting on events of April 1942. We must look elsewhere to highlight the singular achievement of the Great War nurses.

Perhaps it has to do with their ability to nurse on in the face of severe water shortages and debilitating cold. The cold was responsible for countless cases of trench foot, neuritis (nerve inflammation), myalgia (muscle pain), and bronchial pneumonia that the nurses managed. Amputations of toes and feet following weeks lying in the icy slush of trenches were maddeningly common. Sometimes amputation did not await arrival at casualty clearing stations: feet frozen solid simply dropped off during the ambulance rides. Maude Mortimer wrote of "huddled inarticulate bundles of pain and misery with stone cold feet and chatting teeth," whereas Kate Luard simply remarked on soldiers returning on stretchers "starved with cold."[53]

Water shortages were so severe that little was available for scrubbing prior to performing surgery. The cold was so extreme that when a patient's abdomen was opened, steam rose from it. Nurses observing the steam were freezing themselves. In a futile effort to warm up, they wore "fatigues and field jackets under their sterile scrub gowns." But this report does not come from World War I nurses either. The reference to fatigues and scrub gowns gives the game away. We are not in France in 1917 but in South Korea in 1950, and the commentator is army nurse Katherine Jump. Another army nurse, Brigadier General Anna Mae Hays, who served in both World War II and Korea, preferred the steamy jungles of the former to the lack of supplies and lack of warmth of the latter.[54]

Perhaps the singularity of the Great War nurses resides in their ability to cope with mutilating multiple injuries in environments of squalor, rats, mice, lice, fleas, and the absence of antibiotics. In the face of circumstances reported time and again in their letters and diaries, they did not flinch. "Every wound was filthy," recalled one nurse. She beheld boys

> with legs and feet missing, gaping chest and abdominal wounds, and arms barely attached. We used gallons of normal saline to rinse wounds. They were debrided or cleaned out and left open.... Amputees were frequent. A lot of times it wasn't just an arm, but it was more than one limb. They were all young and they look like your kid brother.[55]

Except that the nurse here is Mary Lou Ostergren-Bruner, and she speaks to us not from a casualty clearing station in Flanders but from an evacuation hospital in Pleiku, Vietnam in 1967.

We have dwelt on the multiple ways in which American nurses relied on their hands—as instruments of diagnosis, of consoling attachment, of reassurance, of preparation for lifelong disability or death. Here we strike a more resonant note since, with the advent of antibiotic therapy in World War II, traditional nursing was placed in jeopardy. This, at any rate, is the judgment of Penny Starns, who writes of the quandary of frontline nurses during World War II. How could nurses justify their professional status, she asks, "when one drug could undermine most of their traditional nursing techniques?"[56] Perhaps the remarkably versatile hands of Great War nurses set them apart from nurses whose hands administer antibiotics. There are abundant examples of ameliorative nursing touch at all stages of treatment, recovery, and dying on the Western front. Perhaps the nurses of World War I were simply able to find *time* to reach out and touch their patients, literally, figuratively, emotionally. Was this equally the case for the nurses of World War II and Vietnam? Perhaps antibiotics and new diagnostic and treatment technologies militated again palliative bedside nursing in the Nightingalean tradition:

> We would spend tremendous numbers of hours with the patients, even during our time off. Your shift would be over and there would be guys you realized were just really in agony. We would go over and spend another six or eight hours holding their hand, talking and singing to them, and trying to keep their minds off it until they could have another pain shot.[57]

But here again, we are a half century removed from the trials and tribulations of the Western front. This is the voice of Elizabeth R. Barker, a member of the Navy Nurse Corps caring for Vietnam casualties in a stateside naval hospital in 1967.

Perhaps searching for the singularity of Great War nursing practice alongside that of later wars approaches the issue from the wrong direction. What is striking about the World War I nurses is not the degree to which they differ from but the degree to which they anticipate the nurses of World War II and Vietnam. It is easier to appreciate their achievement by looking back, rather than forward, a half century. Did the nurses of the Civil War prefigure the Great War nurses to the same degree that the latter prefigure the nurses of Vietnam? Civil War nurses were often inspiring caregivers, openly maternal, nurturant, deeply connected with their patients. But their caregiving involved wrangling soldiers' food parcels from corrupt quartermasters and officers and doing everything in their power to keep the boys warm, hydrated, and decently fed. There was little else they could do to promote comfort. Much of their soothing talk and hand holding, moreover, was theological, an effort to ready the wounded for death and the afterlife at a time when wound and postsurgical infections were rampant. The reinfection and death that routinely followed amputation often came quickly, providing little opportunity for the bedside comfort care of prolonged convalescence.

The Civil War nurses cared for their patients in all the ways their historical moment permitted. Yes, there were nurses who did more: Many Union nurses in field hospitals became competent to do dressings and bandaging, and a small number found themselves in operating tents alongside surgeons in the heat of major campaigns. But these nurses were heroic exceptions to the rule, and they were not empowered by the experience. Allowing for brilliant exceptions—Clara Barton, Mary Ellis, Emily Elizabeth Parsons, and others—the nurses were untrained mid-nineteenth-century women volunteers who went to war out of patriotism and an obligation to provide a measure of maternal comfort to the wounded. It followed, especially in the South, that most nurses, Ada Bacot among them, limited their nursing to what was appropriate to woman's sphere, not to what was necessary to save lives.[58] Within this sphere, they assisted doctors primarily by doing laundry, preparing meals, bringing the occasional food treat, and reading and writing letters at bedside. They returned home from the war much as they had set out for it—as untrained women volunteers who grew into their wartime roles, but whose presence on the battlefield was frowned on, especially by Southern surgeons and officers. As such, these nurses, for all their courage and caring, are premodern nurses whose role in the war between the states closed one chapter of military nursing in the United States.

In the Civil War, the nurse's arsenal of wound management, on and off the battlefield, consisted of bandaging, lint, plaster, shears, sponges, and a bottle of chloroform. Nursing skill included the ability to prepare a suitably strong mustard or flax seed poultice.[59] In the pre-bacteriological, pre-antiseptic era, medications deadened pain and nothing more. Chloroform, ether, morphine, and brandy were the staples, available (or not) to surgeons and nurses alike.

The half century that separates the nurses of World War I from their Civil War forbears is the same half century that separates the nurses of World War I from their Vietnam-era descendants. And yet the Great War nurses, with their scalpels and probes; their irrigation tubes and antiseptics; their ability to manage shock, hemorrhage, and respiratory distress; and their mastery of the complicated gas anesthesia machinery, are recognizably modern. Great War nurses understood bacteriology and principles of disease transmission and, in this respect too, are recognizably modern. Civil War nurses lived in the mid-nineteenth-century world of miasmas. Specific technologies separate the nurses of World War I from nurses a half century later, but not the acceptance of technology as integral to nursing care. In 1917, prior to disembarking for France, Helen Fairchild's nursing students give her "a dandy case of instruments" that includes, among other things, a "hypo-syringe," dressing scissors, forceps, a folding scalpel, two probes, a glass catheter, a thermometer, and "a little instrument for taking out foreign bodies." For Emily Parsons, a half century earlier, a bandage roller was an instrument *au courant*, "a most useful little thing."[60]

The American nurses of World War I stand midway between the Civil War and the war in Vietnam. Chronologically they straddled two nursing worlds. What marks them as the originators of modern nursing practice is how little straddling they actually did. Rather they threw themselves across the temporal divide and embraced a thoroughly scientific worldview, and this despite the embryonic modernity that this worldview sustained. They understood the bacterial cause of gas gangrene, but also knew that many of their patients would undergo multiple amputations and still die when their infections entered the blood stream. They understood that Spanish flu was caused by a microorganism of some sort and waited hopefully for lab scientists to develop an effective serum, just as they had for other infectious diseases. They put in long hours monitoring and adjusting Carrel-Dakin drips, understanding the scientific rationale of the treatment but knowing that the system would fail to prevent amputation and death some of the time. They stayed with shell-shocked patients during periods of desperately symptomatic unraveling, providing a therapeutic holding environment that allowed for slow recovery over time. And they stayed with severe burn patients, even when massive internal damage made an agonized death certain. Absent the anti-inflammatories and collagen-based dressings of a later generation, they could do nothing to ease their passing. An aspect of their modernity is how they became conditioned to failure without allowing failure to jeopardize their reliance on science or their hopeful expectation of a better science around the corner—better antiseptics, better irrigation systems, better serums, better surgical techniques, better burn treatments, better devices for fracture management. Their nursing practice was wed to the best science available to them, so that their failures to save patients became, as the British would say, brilliant failures that attested to the limits of their science but not the value of science per se.

World War I nurses rarely took refuge in the type of religious consolation common among the nurses of the Civil War.[61] The attitude that came from a commitment to scientific nursing, deepened when possible by caring touch, is beautifully captured by Kate Luard. Luard, it is true, is a British nursing sister, but her avowal of purpose in the face of horror speaks eloquently to a sense of professionalism that traverses national boundaries. Like the European and Canadian nurses who preceded them, America's Great War nurses fearlessly engaged the worst that modern mechanized warfare threw at them as they marched into a realm of professionalized caregiving that lives on into the present. So here is Kate Evelyn Luard, veteran of the Boer War and the Great War, recipient of the 1st class Royal Red Cross Medal and Bar, writing during the Battle of Arras in the fall of 1916:

> There is no form of horror imaginable, on any part of the human body, that we can't tackle ourselves now, and no extreme of shock or collapse is considered too hopeless to cope with, except the few who die in a few minutes after admission.[62]

Chapter Notes

Chapter 1

1. Shirley Millard, *I Saw Them Die: Diary and Recollections*, ed. Adele Comandini (New York: Harcourt, Brace, 1936), 7.

2. Julia C. Stimson, *Finding Themselves: The Letters of an American Army Chief Nurse in a British Hospital in France* (New York: Macmillan, 1918), 3–4.

3. Helen Fairchild, letters of approx. May 19, 1917, in Nelle Fairchild Hefty Rote, *Nurse Helen Fairchild: WWI 1917–1918* (Lewisburg, PA: privately published, 2004), 35.

4. Fairchild, letter of May 22, 1917, in Rote, *Nurse Helen Fairchild* (ftnt 3), 37.

5. Jane E. Schultz, *Women at the Front: Hospital Workers in Civil War America* (Chapel Hill: University of North Carolina Press, 2004), 46, 49.

6. Fairchild, letter of May 22, 1917, in Rote, *Nurse Helen Fairchild* (ftnt 3), 38–39.

7. Eric Scott, ed., *Nobody Ever Wins a War: The World War 1 Diaries of Ella Mae Bongard, R.N.* (Ottawa: Janeric, 1997), diary entries of October 5, 9, and 12, 1917, 10–12.

8. Stimson, *Letters* (ftnt 2), 3–4; Millard, *I Saw Them Die* (ftnt 1), 7; Shari Lynn Wigle, *Pride of America: The Letters of Grace Anderson, U.S. Army Nurse Corps, World War I* (Rockville, MD: Seaboard, 2007), 9.

9. David M. Kennedy, *Over Here: The First World War and American Society* (Oxford: Oxford University Press, 2004 [1980]), 178–179.

10. Charlotte Dale, "The Social Exploits and Behaviour of Nurses During the Anglo-Boer War, 1899–1902," in Helen Sweet & Sue Hawkins, *Colonial Caring: A History of Colonial and Post-Colonial Nursing* (Manchester: Manchester University Press, 2015), 60–83, at 66–68. This chapter grows out of Dale's unpublished dissertation, *Raising Professional Confidence: The Influence of the Anglo-Boer War (1899–1902) on the Development and Recognition of Nursing as a Profession*, University of Manchester, 2014, 66–92.

11. Dale, *Raising Professional Confidence* (ftnt 10), 93ff. The male orderlies who provided actual nursing care were of variable quality. Some had received training in general nursing duties by the Royal Army Medical Corps; others had attended all of five lectures on nursing as volunteer members of the St. John's Ambulance Brigade; and a final contingent comprised convalescing patients. It followed that the quality of nursing care received by the wounded was very hit-or-miss, with some orderlies extolled for skilled bedside nursing and others accused of murdering patients through neglect (100–103).

12. Jean S. Edmonds, quoted in Philip A. Kalisch, "Heroines of '98: Female

Army Nurses in the Spanish-American War," *Nursing Research*, 24:411–429, 1975, at 414.

13. Amy Wingreen, "The Poor Men Were So Glad to See Me: A War Nurse in Cuba, 1898," *Missouri Review*, 16:97–130, 1993, quoted at 127.

14. See Mark A. D. Howe, comp., *The Occasional Speeches of Justice Oliver Wendell Holmes, Jr.* (Cambridge: Harvard University Press, 1962), 73–80.

15. *The Biblical World*, 49:137–138, March, 1917, at 138.

16. *North Amer. Rev.*, 201:676–682, May, 1915, cited in Michael S. Neiberg, *The Path to War: How the First World War Created Modern America* (New York: Oxford University Press, 2016), 76.

17. This is the thesis of Richard Gamble, persuasively argued and documented in *The War for Righteousness: Progressive Christianity, the Great War, and the Rise of the Messianic Nation* (Wilmington, DE: ISI, 2003). In *Faith in the Fight: Religion and the American Soldier in the Great War* (Princeton: Princeton University Press, 2010), Jonathan Ebel argues, albeit less persuasively, that American soldiers took their religion, especially Christianity, onto the battlefield, where it provided a framework for accepting the chaos, suffering, and death that often awaited them.

18. On the prewar discussion of Jesus as a "manly redeemer," see especially Stephen Prothero, *American Jesus: How the Son of God Became a National Hero* (New York: Farrar, Strauss & Giroux, 2003), 87–123.

19. Ebel, *Faith in the Fight* (ftnt 17), loc 157, 272, 461.

20. Hibben and Herrick, cited in Kennedy, *Over Here* (ftnt 9), 179.

21. According to Cirillo, only 54 American nurses served in both the Spanish-American War and WWI, and these figures result from using "the broadest method of counting." He can identify only 12 nurses who were veterans of both wars, having met the minimum service requirement (90 days) of each war. Vincent J. Cirillo, *Bullets and Bacilli: The Spanish-American War and Military Medicine* (New Brunswick: Rutgers University Press, 2004), 232–233.

22. Kennedy, *Over Here* (ftnt 9), 180.

23. Fairchild, letter of May 26, 1917, in Rote, *Nurse Helen Fairchild* (ftnt 3), 47.

24. Fairchild, letter of approx. May 19, 1917, in Rote, *Nurse Helen Fairchild* (ftnt 3), 34–37; Isabel Anderson, *Zigzagging: An American Female Nurse's Experiences During WWI* (Washington, D.C.: Westphalia, 2015 [1937]), 5; "The Journal of Emma Elizabeth Weaver," in *Nurses of World War One: Service Beyond Expectations*, ed., Lorraine Luciano & Casandra Jewell (Carlisle, PA: Army Heritage Center Foundation, 2006), 17.

25. "Some of them are such infants to be fighting for their country." Kate Luard, *Unknown Warriors: The Letters of Kate Luard, RRC and Bar, Nursing Sister in France, 1914–1918*, ed. John & Caroline Stevens (Stroud: History Press, 2014), loc 307.

26. Edith Appleton, *A Nurse at the Front: The First World War Diaries*, ed. R. Cowen (London: Simon & Schuster UK, 2012), 138; Cirillo, *Bullets and Bacilli* (ftnt 21), letter of July 10, 1917, 67.

27. N. A. (possibly M. E. Clark), *A War Nurse's Diary: Sketches from a Belgian Field Hospital* (New York: Macmillan, 1918), 14.

28. Enid Bagnold, a volunteer nurse (VAD) at London's Royal Herbert Hospital in 1918, wrote of a soldier with 11 wounds, including two smashed arms. See Enid Bagnold, *A Diary Without Dates* (London: Heinemann, 1918), 125.

29. Millard, *I Saw Them Die* (ftnt 1), 152; Appleton, *Nurse at the Front* (ftnt 26), 189.

30. Dorothea Crewdson, *Dorothea's War: A First World War Nurse Tells her Story*, ed. Richard Crewdson (London: Weidenfeld & Nicolson, 2013), 56; Millard, *I Saw Them Die* (ftnt 1), 12; Helen Dore Boylston, *Sister: The War Diary of a Nurse* (s.l.: Kismet, 2018 [1925], 76; Beatrice Hopkinson, *Nursing Through*

Shot & Shell: A Great War Nurse's Story, ed. Vivien Newman (South Yorkshire: Pen & Sword, 2014), 82, 85.

31. Agnes Warner, *'My Beloved Poilus'* (St. John: Barnes, 1917), loc 639; Judith S. Graham, *The World War I Letters of Nora Saltonstall* (Boston: Northeastern University Press, 2004), 179.

32. Bongard, *Diaries* (ftnt 7), 22.

33. Kate Wilson, *Lights Out! The Memoir of Nursing Sister Kate Wilson: Canadian Army Medical Corps, 1915– 1017* (Ottawa: CEF Books, 2004 [1981]), 163.

34. Alice Isaacson, "Diary-1917," Library & Archives, Canada (http://www. bac-lac.gc.ca/eng/discover/military-herit age/first-world-war/canada-nursing-sisters/Pages/alice-isaacson.aspx) letter of December 10, 1917, pp. 102–105.

35. Wilson-Simmie, *Lights Out!* (ftnt 8), 146.

36. *Journal of Emma Elizabeth Weaver* (ftnt 24), entry of January 22, 1919, 222– 223.

37. Sophronia Bucklin, *In Hospital and Camp: A Woman's Record of Thrilling Incidents among the Wounded in the Late War* (Phila: John A. Potter, 1869), 223– 224.

38. Lucille Ross Jones, in Margorie Barron Norris, *Sister Heroines: The Roseate Glow of Wartime Nursing, 1914– 1918* (Calgary: Bunker To Bunker, 2002), 28–29.

39. Isaacson, "Diary-1917" (ftnt 34), pp. 107–108.

40. Boylston, *Diary* (ftnt 30), 37.

41. Mary Borden, *The Forbidden Zone,* ed. H. Hutchison (London: Hesperus, 2008 [1928]), 44.

42. Boylston, *Sister* (ftnt 30), 48.

43. Bagnold, *Diary* (ftnt 28), ebook loc 25, 104; Ellen N. LaMotte, *The Backwash of War: The Human Wreckage of the Battlefield as Witnessed by an American Hospital Nurse* (New York: Putnam's, 1916), 139.

44. Boylston, *Diary* (ftnt 30), 93.

45. Millard, *I Saw Them Die* (ftnt 1), 110–111.

46. All the brief essays in LaMotte's *Backwash of War* (ftnt 43) and Borden's *Forbidden Zone* (ftnt 41) circle around these and related themes. Among them, I was especially moved by LaMotte's "Alone," "Locomotor Ataxia," and "A Surgical Triumph," and Borden's "Rosa," "Paraphernalia," and "In the Operating Room."

47. Christine E. Hallett, *Containing Trauma: Nursing Work in the First World War* (Manchester: Manchester University Press, 2009), 177.

48. I have in mind especially the excellent studies of Christine Hallett, *Containing Trauma* (ftnt 47); *Veiled Warriors: Allied Nurses of the First World War* (Oxford: Oxford University Press, 2014); and *Nurses of Passchendaele: Caring for the Wounded of the Ypres Campaigns, 1914–1918* (South Yorkshire: Pen & Sword, 2017).

49. Kate Cumming, *Kate: The Journal of a Confederate Nurse* (Baton Rouge: Louisiana State University Press, 1959 [1866]), 33.

50. Florence Nightingale, *Notes on Nursing: What Nursing Is, What Nursing Is Not* (London: Harrison, 1859), and widely reprinted in many editions.

51. Bucklin, *In Hospital and Camp* (ftnt 37), 254.

52. *Ibid.,* 270–271.

53. Emily Elizabeth Parsons, *Memoir: Published for the Benefit of the Cambridge Hospital* (Boston: Little, Brown, 1880, 15, 18; Jane E. Schultz, ed., *The Birth Place of Souls: The Civil War Nursing Diary of Harriet Eaton* (Oxford: OUP, 2011), letters of March 18, 1853 and October 16, 1864, 129, 154.

54. Jean V. Berlin, ed., *A Confederate Nurse: The Diary of Ada W. Bacot, 1860– 1863* (Columbia: University of South Carolina Press, 2000), 67.

55. Bucklin, *In Hospital and Camp* (ftnt 37), 259.

56. *Eaton, Diary* (ftnt 53), entries of December 13, 15, 17 & 18, 1862, pp. 91– 93.

57. Parsons, *Memoir* (ftnt 53), 20.

58. Yoshiya Makita, "Professional Angels at War: The United States Army Nursing Service and Changing Ideals of Nursing at the Turn of the Twentieth Century," *Japanese Journal of American Studies*, 24:2013, 67–86.

59. The editors of the *British Medical Journal* were among those skeptical of McGee's accomplishments. Editorializing in April 1905, they claimed on the authority of American journalists "that in fact they [McGee and her nine nurses] were regarded somewhat in the light of white elephants by the Japanese. As they could not speak the language, they were useless in the hospitals. Their presence was an embarrassment and an expense to their hosts as they required separate accommodation and special food. Mrs. McGee seems to think that she accomplished something by lecturing on sick diet…but, on her own showing, the Japanese nurses can do all that American nurses can do and a great deal which they cannot, and they do it all with a minimum of fuss." N.A., "American Nurses in Japan," *Brit. Med. J.*, 1:963–964, 1905.

60. Kalisch, "Heroines of '98" (ftnt 12), 414.

61. Victor C. Vaughan, *A Doctor's Memories* (Indianapolis: Bobbs-Merrill, 1926), 269ff., 286. Further weight was lent to the Commission's finding in 1902, when Robert Koch determined that a typhoid fever epidemic in Trier, Germany was caused by healthy human carriers. Thomas D. Brock, *Robert Koch: A Life in Medicine and Bacteriology* (Washington, D.C.: ASM, 1998 [1988]), 255–256.

62. Gerald J. Pierce, *Public and Private Voices: The Typhoid Fever Experience at Camp Thomas*. Unpublished dissertation, Department of History, Georgia State University, 2007, 166–167, 220–228.

63. Wingreen, "The Poor Men Were So Glad" (ftnt 13), 118.

64. Ann K. Frantz, "Clara Barton in the Spanish-American War," *Amer. J. Nurs.*, 98:39–41, 1998), at 41.

65. Pierce, *Public and Private Voices* (ftnt 62), 219; Fannie Dennie, "The Experience of an Army Nurse," *Trained Nurse Hospital Review*, 22:111–118, 1899.

66. Nicholas Senn, *Medico-Surgical Aspects of the Spanish American War* (Chicago: AMA Press, 1900), 316.

67. *Ibid.*, 56, 318–319.

68. *Ibid.*, 295–296.

69. *Ibid.*, 300–301.

70. Mercedes Graf, *On the Field of Mercy: Women Medical Volunteers from the Civil War to the First World War* (Amherst, NY: Humanity Books, 2010), 229.

71. Helen B. Schuler and Florence M. Kelly, quoted in Kalisch, "Heroines of '98" (ftnt 12), 415.

72. Amanda Akins Stearns, *The Lady Nurse of Ward E, 1863–1864* (New York: Baker & Taylor, 1909), 101.

73. Alice Bron, *Diary of a Nurse in South Africa: Being a Narrative of Experiences in the Boer and English Hospital Service* (London: Chapman & Hall, 1901), 147, 165.

74. Bron spent her first several weeks in South Africa caring for English and Boer typhoid patients in a hospital of only 20 beds occupying a small church in Jacobsdal. *Ibid.*, 31–34.

75. Sister X, *The Tragedy and Comedy of War Hospitals* (New York: Dutton, 1906), 99–100.

76. Georgina Fane Pope, "Nursing in South Africa During the Boer War, 1899–1900," *Amer. J. Nurs.*, 3:10–14, 1902, at 12. Ergot alkaloids are still used to treat migraine headaches and to induce uterine contractions and then control the bleeding that follows childbirth.

77. Sister X, *Tragedy and Comedy* (ftnt 75), 121–122.

78. W. S. Inder, *On Active Service with the S.J.A.B., South African War, 1899–1902* (Kendal: Atkinson and Pollitt, 1903), 55–56, 36.

79. Rodney D. Sinclair & Terence J. Ryan, "A Great War for Antiseptics," *Australas. J. Dermatol.*, 34:115–118, 1993. These nineteenth-century antiseptics in-

cluded salicylic, thymol, Eucalyptus oil, aluminum acetate, and boric acid. The last was widely used in ointment form during the war.

80. Senn, *Medico-Surgical Aspects* (ftnt 66), 106. A report in the *American Journal of Nursing* in 1917 noted that trained nurses had only recently been allowed into the outer fluoroscopy room of the "x-ray laboratory," where they maintained the "bismuth-meal tray" and served patients barium or bismuth "meals," administered enemas for "colonic fillings," and labelled and filed the x-ray plates. See Louise B. D'Arby, "The Hospital X-Ray Nurse," *Amer. J. Nurs.*, 17:488–490, 1917.

81. Nurses through World War I had only the Nightingalean pledge of 1893 to guide them. The American Nursing Association first broached the matter of a code of ethics at its annual convention of 1926, but the question was referred to committee and then put to the readership of the *American Journal of Nursing* in 1928 for reader feedback. It was only in 1950 that the ANA finally adopted a code of ethics for professional nurses in the form of 17 statements. In true Nightingalean fashion, ethical conduct was linked to nurses' obligation "to carry out the physician's orders intelligently, to avoid misunderstandings or inaccuracies by verifying orders, and to refuse to participate in unethical procedures." See L. Freitas, "Historical Roots and Future Perspectives Related to Nursing Ethics," *J. Prof. Nurs.*, 197–205, 1990.

82. The VAD (Voluntary Aid Detachment) program was founded in 1909 to provide nurses' aides to British military hospitals. Canada also had a smaller VAD program, with all Canadian VADs trained and certified by St. John Ambulance Association and assigned either to Canadian Convalescent hospitals or British military hospitals. In this book, I choose not to characterize VADs as aides, since they did receive several months of training and had to pass exams and receive certifications in first aid and home nursing. Moreover, the shortage of graduate nurses meant that, in many field and base hospitals, senior VADs grew into, and assumed the responsibilities of, graduate nurses. They are closer to what Americans think of as "practical nurses" who, upon receiving licenses, become L.P.N.s (licensed practical nurses). In the chapters to follow, I usually refer to V.A.D.s, following the practice of other historians, as voluntary nurses. In British and Canadian military hospitals, they addressed them as "Nurse" whereas graduate nurses were always addressed as "Sisters."

Chapter 2

1. Frances Cluett, *Your Daughter Fanny: War Letters of Frances Cluett, VAD*, ed. Bill Rompkey & Bert Riggs (St. John's NL: Flanker, 2006), letter of March 31, 1918, 148.

2. http://thebiglead.com/2015/11/18/fanduel-draftkings-commercials-new-york-attorney general; https://www.realclearpolitics.com/2018/06/28/demo crats_are_in_the_middle_of_a_blood bath_446146.html; https://www.huffin-gtonpost.in/2017/05/12/indian-it-work-ers-brace-for-bloodbath-as-industry-veers-towards_a_22082707.

3. Beatrice Hopkinson, *Nursing through Shot & Shell: A Great War Nurse's Story*, ed. Vivien Newman (South Yorkshire: Pen & Sword, 2014), ebook loc 1434; N.A., *A War Nurse's Diary: Sketches from a Belgian Field Hospital* (Cornwall, UK: Diggory, 2005 [1918]), ebook loc 805–820.

4. N.A., *Diary* [ftnt 3], 19.

5. On triaging, see for example Nelle Fairchild Hefty Rote, *Nurse Helen Fairchild, WWI 1917–1918* (Lewisburg, PA: privately printed, 2004), letter of August 14, 1917), 139. Cf. Christine E. Hallett, *Nurses of Passchendaele: Caring for the Wounded of the Ypres Campaigns*, 1914–1918 (South Yorkshire: Pen & Sword, 2017), 101, 110.

6. Maude Essig, "My Trip Abroad with Uncle Sam, 1917–1919" (Maude Essig World War I Diary), Illinois Wes-

leyan Historical Collections, entry of July 27, 1918, at 44.

7. George Crile, *An Autobiography*, vol 1, ed. Grace Crile (Phila: Lippincott, 1947), 68–69. 72, 75.

8. Elizabeth Rosanna Bundy, *Surgical Nursing in War* (Phila: Blakiston, 1917), 31.

9. J. E. Cossnett, "The Origins of Intravenous Fluid Therapy," *Lancet*, 333:768–771, 1989; Thomas F. Baskett, "William O'Shaughnessy, Thomas Latta and the Origins of Intravenous Saline," *Resuscitation*, 55:231–234, 2002.

10. Greater use was made—also for the first time—of heated water beds to warm patients and help prevent shock. See Richard A. Gabriel, *Between Flesh and Steel: A History of Military Medicine from the Middle Ages to the War in Afghanistan* (Washington, D.C.: Potomac, 2013), 199.

11. Bundy, *Surgical Nursing* (ftnt 8), 36.

12. Among the few references to blood transfusion among the nurses, see Shirley Millard, *I Saw Them Die: Diary and Recollections*, ed. Adele Comandini (New York: Harcourt, Brace, 1936), 83 and Isabel Anderson, *Zigzagging: An American Female Nurse's Experience during WWI* (Washington, D.C.: Westphalia, 2015 [1918]), 59.

13. Crile, *Autobiography* (ftnt 7), 165–167. The prehistory of blood transfusion in its scientific, cultural, and religious aspects is engagingly told in Holly Tucker, *Blood Work: A Tale of Medicine and Murder in the Scientific Revolution* (New York: Norton, 2012).

14. Crile, *Autobiography* (ftnt 7), 256.

15. Robertson was invited to British field hospitals to teach transfusion technique; he also showed how citrated blood collected from Type O (universal) donors could be stored and shipped.

16. Julia C. Stimson, *Finding Themselves: The Letters of an American Army Chief Nurse in a British Hospital in France* (New York: Macmillan, 1918), 123.

17. Eusol was an antiseptic solution prepared from chlorinated lime and boric acid, formerly used in treating wounds.

18. Quoted in Rote, *Nurse Helen Fairchild* (ftnt 5), 125.

19. Helen Dore Boylston, *Sister: The War Diary of a Nurse* (New York: Washburn, 1927), entry of 27 March 1918, 39.

20. Stimson, *Finding Themselves* (ftnt 16), 142.

21. [Kate Norman Derr], *"Mademoiselle Miss": Letters from an American Girl Serving with the Rank of Lieutenant in a French Army Hospital at the Front* (Boston: Butterfield, 1916), 21.

22. May Tilton Memoir, quoted in Hallett, *Nurses of Passchendaele* (ftnt 5), 146.

23. "One morning in 1908 while making rounds I drew Miss Hodgins aside and presented to her what amounted to an annunciation. She had received no warning whatever about the plan to make her my special anesthetist, but she told me promptly that she would undertake it if I would remember always that she was giving her best. This was the beginning of the first school of anesthesia in the world." Crile, *Autobiography* (ftnt 7), 195.

24. In her history of anesthesia, Virginia Thatcher quotes Arthur Dean Bevan in 1917 that: "Women...make the best anesthetists just as they make the most reliable and conscientious operating-room nurses. In these days of modern surgery, the responsibilities and the functions of the skilled anesthetist and the head surgical nurse are little less important than those of the operator himself" (Virginia S. Thatcher, *History of Anesthesia, With Emphasis on the Nurse Specialist* [Philadelphia: Lippincott, 1953], 76).

25. *Ibid.*, 95.

26. In 1906 Magaw reported over 14,000 cases of open-drop anesthesia without a single death directly attributable to the anesthesia. See Marianne Bankert, *Watchful Care: A History of America's Nurse Anesthetists* (New York: Continuum, 1989), 131 and Bruce Evan

Koch, "Surgeon-Nurse Anesthetist Collaboration Advanced Surgery Between 1889 and 1950,"*Anathesia-Analgesia,* 12:653–662, 2015, at 654.

27. Harvey Cushing, journal entry of 3 August 1917, quoted in Michael Bliss, *Harvey Cushing: A Life in Surgery* (Oxford: OUP, 2005), 123. Interestingly, the passage mentioning Garrard is omitted from the 3 August 1917 entry in the 1936 edition of Cushing's journal, *From a Surgeon's Journal, 1915–1918* (Boston: Little, Brown, 1936), at 177. Cushing mentions "Miss Garrard" elsewhere in his journal as a member of his mobile surgical team (152,161, 180, 254).

28. Martin Ramon, "Anesthesia at Base Hospital No. 5," presented at the 9th International Symposium on the History of Anesthesia, Boston, MA, 2017.

29. s.n., *History of the Pennsylvania Hospital Unit (Base Hospital No. 10, USA)* (New York: Hoeber, 1921), 57, 93; Koch, "Surgeon-Nurse Anesthetist Collaboration" (ftnt 26), 658.

30. Thatcher, *History of Anesthesia* (ftnt 24), 100.

31. *Ibid.*, 99, 97.

32. Alma A. Clarke, "Notebook," in Alma A. Clarke Papers, 1914–1946, Special Collections Department, Bryn Mawr College Library, Bryn Mawr, PA.

33. Mary Ellis, "Reminiscences," in Mary Gardner Holland, *Our Army Nurses: Stories from Women in the Civil War* (Roseville, MN: Edinborough, 1998 [1895], 87–89, at 87.

34. Elizabeth Brown Pryor, *Clara Barton: Professional Angel* (Philadelphia: University of Pennsylvania Press, 1988), 99; Stephen B. Oates, *A Woman of Valor: Clara Barton and the Civil War* (New York: Free Press, 1994), 86.

35. Emily Elizabeth Parsons, *Memoir, Published for the Benefit of the Cambridge Hospital* (Cambridge: John Wilson, 1880), 134.

36. *Ibid.*, 23.

37. Gabriel, *Between Flesh and Steel* (ftnt 10), 195.

38. *Ibid.*, 200.

39. Alice Bron, *Diary of a Nurse in South Africa: Being a Narrative of Experiences in the Boer and English Hospital Service* (London: Chapman & Hall, 1901), 32, 63.

40. Among many examples are Edith Appleton, *A Nurse at the Front: The First World War Diaries*, ed. R. Cowen (London: Simon & Schuster UK, 2012), 161, 203; Boylston, *Diary* (ftnt 19), 37; Derr, *"Mademoiselle Miss"* (ftnt 21), entry of 24 March 1918, 33.

41. A. Carrel and G. Dehelly, *The Treatment of Infected Wounds*, trans. Herbert Child (New York: Hoeber, 1917), 4. Another criticism of the Carrel-Dakin method, made by Almroth Wright in particular, was that the microbes were inaccessible to antiseptics because they lay on the "inner face of a torn and ragged track; and that track is blocked by blood clot and hernia of muscle" (Sir A. E. Wright, "An Address on Wound Infections; and on Some New Methods for the Study of the Various Factors Which Come into Consideration in Their Treatment," *Proc. R. Soc. Med.*, 8:41–86, 1915, at 68).

42. Carrel & Dehelly (ftnt 41), 22.

43. *Ibid.*, 13.

44. *Ibid.*, 20. The two chemicals used to neutralize the hypochlorite (i.e., to eliminate its free alkali) were hypochlorous acid and boric acid (22).

45. *Ibid.*, 23.

46. William O'Neill Sherman, "The Abortive Treatment of Wound Infection: Carrel's Method—Dakin's Solution," *JAMA*, 69:185–192, 1917, at 187. On Daufresne's refinement of the formula, which concerned the ratios for combining the bleach solution with sodium carbonate and sodium bicarbonate, see also Bundy, *Surgical Nursing in War* (ftnt 8), 42.

47. Carrel & Dehelly (ftnt 31), 15–16.

48. *Ibid.*, 14, 23.

49. Max Bornstein, "Aids in the Use of Dakin-Carrel Treatment," *JAMA*, 70:1820, 1918. For a fuller presentation of Carrel-Dakin treatment—the appara-

tus, the method, and the reasons for its effectiveness—aimed expressly at battlefield nurses, see Bundy, *Surgical Nursing* (ftnt 8), 42.

50. Hallett, *Nurses of Passchendaele* (ftnt 5), 92.

51. Here I follow Dakin's own summary description of the precautions involved in using Carrel's apparatus, in Henry Drysdale Dakin & Edward Kellogg Dunham, *A Handbook on Antiseptics* (New York: Macmillan, 1917), 13–14.

52. Dakin gives the concentration of the solution as either 0.5 percent or as 0.45 to 0.5 percent. *Ibid.*, 13, 23, quoted at 23. On the preparation of the tubing, see, e.g., Anderson, *Zigzagging* (ftnt 12), 130.

53. E. M. Pilcher & A. J. Hull, "The Treatment of Wounds by Flavine," *BMJ*, i(2908):172, 1918.

54. J. S. Dunne, "Notes on Surgical Work in a General Hospital—With Special Reference to the Carrel-Dakin Method of Treatment," *BMJ*, 2:283–284, 1918 is especially laudatory of the Sisters, whose "careful attention to detail largely contributed to the success obtained in the use of Carrel-Dakin method" (284).

55. Derr, "Mademoiselle Miss" (ftnt 21), 20–21. Prior to America's entry into the war, Tuffier, along with the Belgian surgeon Antoine Depage, had extended the Carrel-Dakin method to the treatment of empyema "with much success." In this application, according to the British military surgeon Anthony Bowlby, "The various diverticula [tubular sacs branching off the lining of, in this instance, the pleural cavity] were traced by x-ray pictures of the chest by the introduction of the rubber tubes threated with silver wire." Anthony A. Bowlby, letter to W. W. Keen, in W. W. Keen, *The Treatment of War Wounds* (Phila: Saunders, 1917), 132.

56. Nancy Wagner, ed., *Alice in France: The World War I letters of Alice M. O'Brien* (St. Paul, MN: Minnesota Historical Society Press, 2017), letter of June 3, 1918, 63–68; Anderson, *Zigzagging* (ftnt 12), 12, 130; Emma Elizabeth

Weaver, *The Journal of Emma Elizabeth Weaver*, ed. Lorraine Luciano & Casandra Jewell (Carlisle, Pa: Army Heritage Center Foundation, 2006), 49 [198].

57. Ella Mae Bongard, *Nobody Ever Wins a War: The World War I Diaries of Ella Mae Bongard, R.N.*, ed. Eric Scott (Ottawa: Janeric, 1997), letter of December 1, 1917, 23.

58. Anderson, *Zigzagging* (ftnt 12), 130.

59. E.M.W., "Letters from Nurses in Service," *Amer. J. Nurs.*, 69:715–718, 1919.

60. Christine E. Hallett, *Containing Trauma: Nursing Work in the First World War* (Manchester: Manchester University Press, 2009), 56–59, 46. Anyone writing about nursing in World War I owes an enormous debt to Hallett, whose three exemplary studies, *Containing Trauma* (op. cit.); *Veiled Warriors: Allied Nurses of the First World War* (New York: OUP, 2014); and *Nurses of Passchendaele* (ftnt 5) provide additional examples of some of the nursing activities addressed in this chapter, albeit focusing on the nurses of Britain and the British Dominions.

61. Ellis, "Reminiscences" (ftnt 33), 87; Parsons, *Memoir* (ftnt 35), 48–49, 143.

62. Nancy Josephine Klase, letter of December 2, 1918, "MC 227. World War I Materials, 1918–1919," Barbara Bates Center for the Study of the History of Nursing, University of Pennsylvania School of Nursing.

63. Sarah McNaughtan, *A Woman's Diary of the War: Life of a Nurse at the Front* (New York: Dutton, 1916), 23.

64. Appleton, *Diaries* (ftnt 40), 203; Anderson, *Zigzagging* (ftnt 12), 131; Millard, *I Saw Them Die* (ftnt 12), 15.

65. "Sophie Hoerner Letters," letter of May 10, 1915, Library & Archives of Canada (http://www.bac-lac.gc.ca/eng/discover/military-heritage/first-world-war/canada-nursing-sisters/Pages/sophie-hoerner.aspx). The case that moved Hoerner to tears was of "a young man that had to lose both arms, had a thigh wound, and head."

66. Lucile Rose Jones, quoted in Mar-

jorie Barron Norris, ed., *Sister Heroines: The Roseate Glow of Wartime Nursing, 1914–1919* (Calgary: Bunker to Bunker Publishing, 2002), 26–27.

67. Millard, *I Saw Them Die* (ftnt 12), 13.

68. I discuss this politically charged question and answer it in the affirmative in Paul E. Stepansky, *In the Hands of Doctors: Touch and Trust in Medical Care* (Santa Barbara: Praeger, 2016), 201–225.

Chapter 3

1. [Kate Norman Derr], *"Mademoiselle Miss": Letters from an American Girl Serving with the Rank of Lieutenant in a French Army Hospital at the Front*, preface by Richard C. Cabot (Boston: Butterfield, 1916), 21.

2. *Ibid.*, 67.

3. Helen Dore Boylston, *Sister: The War Diary of a Nurse* (New York: Ives Washburn, 1927), 237.

4. Agnes Warner, *'My Beloved Poilus'* (St. John: Barnes, 1917), 47, cf. 39, 55.

5. Guilhelmi Fabricius Hildanus, *De Gangraena et Sphacelo: Tractatus Methodicus* (Cologne, 1593); J.-G. Maisonneuve & H. Montanier, *Traité pratique des Maladies Vénériennes* (Paris: Labé, 1853).

6. Shauna Devine, *Learning from the Wounded: The Civil War and the Rise of American Medical Science* (Chapel Hill: University of North Carolina Press, 2014), 100–101.

7. *Ibid.*, 102–103.

8. Goldsmith used the term "antiseptic"—which had been in common usage since the 1820s—in its descriptive pre-Listerian sense, viz., as "agents" that promoted the drainage of wounds by breaking up "putrescent" (i.e., decaying) matter. This was an empirical finding that antedated germ theory, which provided an explanation of how and why antiseptics had this effect on wounds. See M. Goldsmith, *A Report on Hospital Gangrene, Erysipelas: As Observed in the Departments of the Ohio and the Cumberland, with Cases Appended, and Pyemia*, published by permission of the surgeon general U.S.A. (Louisville: Bradley & Gilbert, 1863), 16.

9. *Ibid.*, 23, 29–30.

10. See George Thompson, "Battlefield Medicine: The American Response to Gas Gangrene on the Western Front" (https://history.army.mil/curriculum/wwi/docs/AdditionalResources/presentations/GThompson_BM-American_Response_to_Gas_Gangrene.pdf), 7–8, and the government report cited in footnotes 36 & 37.

11. Christine Debue-Barazer, "La gangrène gazeuse pendant la Première Guerre mondiale (Front occidental), *Annales de Démographie Historique*, 1[103] :51–70, 2002, quoted at 68. In the 2012 edition of the *Encyclopedia of Intensive Care Medicine*, ed. Jean-Louis Vincent & Jesse B. Hall (Berlin: Springer-Verlag, 2012), the entry for gas gangrene is given under "Soft tissue infections, Life-Threatening." The entry echoes Debue-Barazer in concluding: "Finally, despite an early diagnosis and appropriate treatment, some patients will lose limbs and others may succumb to systemic complications of the infection."

12. Warner, *Beloved Poilus* (ftnt 4), 103. Cf. Ellen N. La Motte, *The Backwash of War: The Human Wreckage of the Battlefield as Witnessed by an American Hospital Nurse* (New York: Putnam's, 1916), 51.

13. Clare Gass, *War Diary, 1915–1918*, ed. Susan Mann (Montreal: McGill-Queen's University Press, 2000), diary entry of 24 October 1916, 147.

14. Marie Van Horst, *War Letters of an American Woman* (New York: John Lane, 1916), 107–108.

15. Shirley Millard, *I Saw Them Die: Diary and Recollections*, ed. Adele Comandini (New York: Harcourt Brace, 1936), 80.

16. Van Horst, *War Letters* (ftnt 14), 110.

17. "A Canadian Nurse in France," *Amer. J. Nurs.*, 17:790–791, June 1917, at 790.

18. Edith Appleton, *A Nurse at the Front: The First World War Diaries*, ed. R. Cowen (London: Simon & Schuster UK, 2012), 194–195, 240; Beatrice Hopkinson, *Nursing through Shot & Shell: A Great War Nurse's Story*, ed. Vivien Newman (South Yorkshire: Pen & Sword, 2014), 14.

19. Millard, *I Saw Them Die* (ftnt 15), 19.

20. Isabel Anderson, *Zigzagging: An American Female Nurse's Experience during WWI* (Washington, D.C.: Westphalia, 2015 [1918]), 11.

21. Kate Luard, *Unknown Warriors: The Letters of Kate Luard, RRC and Bar, Nursing Sister in France 1914–1918*, ed. John & Caroline Stevens (Stroud: History Press, 117–119, 124.

22. *Ibid.*, 118–119.

23. Derr, *"Mademoiselle Miss"* (ftnt 1), 174ff.

24. Luard, *Letters* (ftnt 21), 30. Sadly "the Prince of Wales" died several days later.

25. Derr, *"Mademoiselle Miss"* (ftnt 1), 47.

26. Luard, *Letters* (ftnt 21), 150.

27. Appleton, *Nurse at the Front* (ftnt 18), 161.

28. Hopkinson, *Nursing through Shot & Shell* (ftnt 18), 65.

29. No less a Civil War nurse than Sophronia Bucklin wrote of "little slender maggots from which a woman's hand is wont to shrink in nervous terror." Sophronia Bucklin, *In Hospital and Camp in the American Civil War* (s.l.: s.n., 2016 [1869], ebook loc 2448.

30. Kosta Y. Mumcuoglu, "Clinical Applications for Maggots in Wound Care," *Amer. J. Clin. Dermatol.*, 4:219–227, 2001, at 225.

31. Millard, *I Saw Them Die* (ftnt 15), 79–80.

32. W. S. Baer, "The Treatment of Chronic Osteomyelitis with the Maggot (larva of the blow fly)," *J. Bone Joint Surg.*, 13:438–475, 1931.

33. The deterrent effect of the "yuck factor" among hospital nurses in Britain has been documented in the doctoral research of the nurse practitioner Sarah Styles. See Frances Robinson, "Maggot Therapy for Wound Healing," *Wound Care*, 12 February 2010, 28–29. The yuck factor has been reduced by shipping and applying live larvae in nylon mesh bags from which they are obscured from view and cannot escape. See Martin Grassberger & Wim Fleischmann, "The Biobag—A New Device for the Application of Medicinal Maggots," *Dermatology* (Basel), 204:306, 2002.

34. There is a large literature on maggot therapy (MDT), from which the following provide a good starting point: Iain S. Whitaker, et al., "Larval therapy from Antiquity to the Present Day: Mechanisms of Action, Clinical Applications and Future Potential," *Postgrad. Med. J.*, 83:409–413, 1980; Kosten Y. Mumcuoglu, "Clinical Applications for Maggots in Wound Care," *Amer. J. Clin. Dermatol.*, 2:219–227, 2001; and Ronald A. Sherman, "Maggot Therapy Takes Us Back to the Future of Wound Care: New and Improved Maggot Therapy for the 21st Century," *J. Diabetes Sci. & Tech.*, 3:336–339, 2009.

35. On Florschütz's invention of the Balkan frame and its use in WWI, see Andrea Emilio Salvi, et al., "The Invention of the Balkan Beam Frame," *Injury, Int. J. Care Injured*, 40:1237–1238, 2009 and Stella Fatović-Ferenčić & Mark Pećina, "The Balkan Beam—Florschütz frame and its Use During the Great War," *Int. Orthopaedics*, 38:2209–2213, 2009. Florschütz's other noteworthy contributions to World War I medicine, which include the adaptation of skull trepanation to the battlefield and the first laparotomies (opening up the abdomen) performed in field hospitals for gunshot and blast wounds, are summarized by Roman Pavic, "Prof. Vatroslav Florschütz and the Balkan Beam Frame," *Injury*, 42:225–226, 2011.

36. Allice Isaacson, "Diary-1917," Library & Archives, Canada (http://www.bac-lac.gc.ca/eng/discover/military-

heritage/first-world-war/canada-nursing-sisters/Pages/alice-isaacson.aspx), letter of December 10, 1917, 102–105.

37. E.g., John Wood, "On the Employment of Double Extension in Cases of Disease and injuries of the Spine and Pelvic Joints," *BMJ*, 1(1014):837–838, 1880; A. R. Jenkins, "The Padded Board Stretcher in the Treatment of Hip Disease and Various Traumata," 8:105–109, 1888; V. Bardenheuer, *The Uses of Permanent Extension: Subcutaneous and Compound Fractures and Dislocations of the Extremities and Their Consequences* (New York: Stechert, 1889); John B. Roberts, Treatment of the Lower End of the Humerus and of the Base of the Radius," *Ann. Surg.*, 16:1–41, 1892, at 28.

38. Elizabeth Bundy, *Surgical Nursing in War* (Phila: Blakiston, 1917), 74–75.

39. Marion G. Parsons, "Some Points in the Nursing of Fractured Femur in the Home," *Amer. J. Nurs.*, 9:104–111, 1908, at 105.

40. Derr, *"Mademoiselle Miss"* (ftnt 1), 95–96.

41. See "She Helps the Wounded," *The Woman Citizen: The Woman's Journal*, 1:431, 3 November 1917. Also Anderson, *Zigzagging* (ftnt 20), 12–13.

42. Hopkinson, *Nursing through Shot & Shell* (ftnt 18), 67.

43. *Plus ça change, plus c'est la même chose*. See Ann Jones's graphic description of the work of these specialists in Mortuary Affairs in *They Were Soldiers: How the Wounded Return from America's Wars—The Untold Story* (Chicago: Haymarket, 2013), chapter 1 ("Secrets: The Dead").

44. Hopkinson, *Nursing through Shot & Shell* (ftnt 18), 67, 70.

45. Mary Borden, *The Forbidden Zone* (London: Hesperus, [1928] 2008), 95–96.

46. Luard, *Letters* (ftnt 21), 39.

47. Van Horst, *Letters* (ftnt 14), 131.

48. Van Horst, *Letters* (ftnt 14), 108.

49. Millard, *I Saw Them Die* (ftnt 15), 15.

50. Bundy, *Surgical Nursing in War* (ftnt 38), 34.

51. Luard, *Letters* (ftnt 21), 72.

52. Millard, *I Saw Them Die* (ftnt 15), 59, 111–112.

53. Maude Mortimer, *A Green Tent in Flanders* (Garden City: Doubleday, Page, 1918), 132–133.

54. Boylston, *Diary* (ftnt 3), loc 534.

55. Millard, *I Saw them Die* (ftnt 15), 109.

56. Dorothea Crewdson, *Dorothea's War: A First World War Nurse Tells Her Story,* ed. Richard Crewdson (London: Weidenfeld & Nicolson, 2013), 51.

57. Sister X, *The Tragedy and Comedy of War Hospitals* (New York: Dutton, 1906), 63–64.

58. Alice Bron, *Diary of a Nurse in South Africa: Being a Narrative of Experiences in the Boer and English Hospital Service*, trans. G. A. Raper (London: Chapman, 1901), 37.

59. Winnicott's notion of "holding" was set forth in many papers during the 1960s, of which the most important are "The Theory of the Parent-Infant Relationship" (1960) and "Dependence in Infant-Care, in Child-Care, and in the Psychoanalytic Setting" (1963), both reprinted in D. W. Winnicott, *The Maturational Processes and the Facilitating Environment: Studies in the Theory of Emotional Development* (New York: International Universities Press, 1965), 37–55 & 249–259.

60. Bucklin, *In Hospital and Camp* (ftnt 29), 269.

61. Emily Elizabeth Parsons, *Memoir* (Boston: Little, Brown, 1880), 77.

62. *Ibid.*, 79, 91.

63. *Ibid.*, 111.

64. See for example S. J. Weiss, "The Language of Touch," *Nurs. Res.*, 28:76–80, 1979; S. J. Weiss, "Psychophysiological Effects of Caregiver Touch on Incidence of Cardiac Dysrhythmia," *Heart Lung*, 15:494–505, 1986; C. A. Estabrooks, "Touch in Nursing Practice: A Historical Perspective: 1900–1920," *J. Nurs. Hist.*, 2:33–49, 1987; J. S. Mulaik, et al., "Patients' Perceptions of Nurses' Use of Touch," *Western. J. Nurs. Res.*,

13:306–323, 1991; J. L. Bottorff, Nurse-Patient Interaction: Observations of Touch (Unpublished Doctoral Dissertation, University of Alberta, 1992), 54–67; C. A. Estabrooks & J. M. Morse, "Toward a Theory of Touch: The Touching Process and Acquiring a Touching Style," *J. Adv. Nurs.*, 17:448–456, 1992; A Carter & H. Sanderson, "The Use of Touch in Nursing Practice," *Nurs. Standard*, 9:31–35, 1995. For a general discussion of the role of tools and touch in medicine and nursing, see Paul E. Stepansky, *In the Hands of Doctors: Touch and Trust in Medical Care* (Santa Barbara: Praeger, 2016), 81–105.

65. On the "good death" as a conduit to the Christian afterlife during the Civil War, see especially Drew Gilpin Faust, *This Republic of Suffering: Death and the American Civil War* (New York: Random House, 2008), 3–31.

66. Sullivan's post–World War II lectures of 1946–1947 were edited and published as Harry Stack Sullivan, *The Interpersonal Theory of Psychiatry*, ed. Helen Swick Perry & Mary Ladd Gawel (New York: Norton, 1953). On "selective inattention," see 319–320, 346–347, 374.

67. Alice Fitzgerald, "To Nurses Preparing for Active Service," *Amer. J. Nurs.*, 18:188–191, 1917, quoted at 189.

68. Van Horst, *War Letters* (ftnt 14), 116.

69. Quoted passage from Crewdson, *Dorothea's War* (ftnt 56), 236–237; also Hopkinson, *Nursing through Shot & Shell* (ftnt 18), 65–67; Isaacson, "Diary 1917" (ftnt 36), entry of 19 June 1918.

70. Luard, *Letters* (ftnt 21), 111; Van Horst, *War Letters* (ftnt 14), 71.

71. Borden, *Forbidden Zone* (ftnt 45), 83; Derr, *"Mademoiselle Miss"* (ftnt 1), 47; Luard, *Letters* (ftnt 21), 121.

Chapter 4

1. Maude Frances Essig, *My Trip Abroad with Uncle Sam, 1917–1919: How We Won World War I*, unpublished journal written during the summer, 1919,

Tate Archives, Illinois Wesleyan University, entry of March 23, 1918.

2. Guy R. Hasegawa, "Proposals for Chemical Weapons during the American Civil War," *Mil. Med.*, 173:499–506, 208.

3. Haber's military role in WWI, especially his creation of chlorine gas in the service of the fatherland, is well covered in chapter 7 of Detrich Stoltzenberg's comprehensive biography of Haber, published in German in 1994 and translated into English as *Fritz Haber: Chemist, Nobel Laureate, German Jew* (Lexington, MA: Plunkett Lake, 2015). For a breezier but still informative treatment, see Daniel Charles, *Master Mind: The Rise and Fall of Fritz Haber, the Nobel Laureate Who Launched the Age of Chemical Warfare* (New York: HarperCollins, 2005), 141ff., especially 154–165.

4. Edmund Russell, *War and Nature: Fighting Humans and Insects with Chemicals From World War I to Silent Spring* (Cambridge: Cambridge University Press, 2001), 27–28.

5. C. G. Hurst, et al., "Vesicants," in M.K. Lenhart & S. D. Tuorinsky, eds., *Medical Aspects of Chemical Warfare* (Washington, D.C.: Office of The Surgeon General, 2008), 259–311.

6. Christine E. Hallett, *Veiled Warriors: Allied Nurses of the First World War* (Oxford: OUP, 2014), 79–80, 203.

7. Yuruk Iyriboz, "A Recent Exposure to Mustard Gas in the United States: Clinical Findings of a Cohort (n = 247) 6 Years After Exposure," *MedGenMed*, 6:4, 2004; Eric Laurent Maranda, et al., "Chemical Warfare's Most Notorious Agent Against the Skin," *JAMA Dermatology*, 152:933, 2016.

8. E.g., Julia C. Stimson, *Finding Themselves: The Letters of an American Army Chief Nurse in a British Hospital in France* (New York: Macmillan, 1918), 80; Kate Luard, *Unknown Warriors: The Letters of Kate Luard, RRC and Bar, Nursing Sister in France 1914–1918*, ed. John & Caroline Stevens (Stroud: History Press, 2014), 132–133.

9. Essig, *My Trip Abroad with Uncle*

Sam (ftnt 1), entries of March 30 and June 25, 1918. Passages from Essig's diary, including the entry of March 30, 1918 also appear in Alma S. Woolley, "Hoosier Nurses in France: The World War I Diary of Maude Frances Essig," *Indiana Magazine of History*, 82:37–68, 1986; Vera Brittain, *Testament of Youth* (New York: Penguin, 2005 [1933]), 370.

10. Helen Fairchild, letter of July 18, 1917, in Nelle Fairchild Hefty Rote, *Nurse Helen Fairchild: WWI 1917–1918* (Lewisburg, PA: privately published, 2004), 79.

11. Christine E. Hallett, *Nurses of Passchendaele: Caring for the Wounded of the Ypres Campaigns, 1914–1918* (South Yorkshire: Pen & Sword, 2017), 112.

12. The Canadian nurse Sophie Hoerner, serving with No. 1 Canadian General Hospital in Étaples in 1915, wrote home that the gassed patients "were terrible to see. It's impossible to supply the demand for respirators." Letter of June 4, 1915, Library & Archives, Canada (http://www.bac-lac.gc.ca/eng/discover/military-heritage/first-world-war/canada-nursing-sisters/Pages/sophie-hoerner.aspx).

13. Fairchild, letter of July 18, 1917, in Rote, *Nurse Helen Fairchild* (ftnt 10), 80.

14. Marie and Anselm Chomel, *Red Cross Chapter at Work* (Indianapolis: Hollenbeck, 1920), 254. Base Hospital 32 was the Indianapolis Base Hospital underwritten by Eli Lilly and Company.

15. *Ibid.*, 255–256; Essig, *My Trip Abroad with Uncle Sam* (ftnt 1), entry of March 24, 1918.

16. N. A. (possibly M. E. Clark), *A War Nurse's Diary: Sketches from a Belgian Field Hospital* (New York: Macmillan, 1918), 98–99.

17. Shirley Millard, *I Saw Them Die: Diary and Recollections*, ed. Adele Comandini (New York: Harcourt Brace, 1936), 108.

18. Frances Cluett, *Your Daughter Fanny: War Letters*, ed. Bill Rompkey & Bert Riggs (St. John's, NL, Canada: Flanker, 2006), 113.

19. Clare Gass, *The War Diary of Clare Gass, 1915–1918*, ed. Susan Mann (Montreal: McGill-Queen's University Press, 2000), 116, 126; Luard, *Letters* (ftnt 8), 97; Brittain, *Testament of Youth* (ftnt 9), 360; Helen Dore Boylston, *Sister: The War Diary of a Nurse* (New York: Washburn, 1927), entry of February 23, 1918, 21.

20. Edith Appleton, *A Nurse at the Front: The First World War Diaries of Sister Edith Appleton*, ed., Ruth Cowen (London: Simon & Schuster, 2012), 35–36.

21. Cluett, *War Letters* (ftnt 18), 114.

22. Essig, *My Trip with Uncle Sam* (ftnt 1), entry of March 24, 1918.

23. Erysipelas is an acute bacterial infection of the upper dermis, usually of the arms, legs, and/or face, that is accompanied by red swollen rashes. Without antibiotic treatment, it can spread through the blood stream and cause sepsis.

24. Appleton, *Diaries* (ftnt 20), 111.

25. Rodney D. Sinclair & Terence J. Ryan, "A Great War for Antiseptics," *Australas. J. Dermatol*, 34:115–118, 1993. These nineteenth-century antiseptics included salicylic, thymol, Eucalyptus oil, aluminum acetate, and boric acid. The last was widely used in ointment form during the war.

26. Cluett, *War Letters* (ftnt 18), 132–134; Alma Clarke, "Training Notebook of 1914," Alma A. Clarke Papers, 1914–1946, Special Collections Department, Bryn Mawr College Library.

27. Boylston, *Diary* (ftnt 19), 19.

28. Kathleen Yarwood (VAD, Dearnley Military Hospital), in Lyn MacDonald, *The Roses of No Man's Land* (London: Penguin, 1993 [1980]), 197–198.

29. Luard, *Letters* (ftnt 8), 88.

30. Agnes Warner, *My Beloved Poilus* (St. John: Barnes, 1917), 70, 86.

31. *Ibid.*, 122.

32. Millard (ftnt 17), *I Saw Them Die*, 108.

33. [Kate Norman Derr], *"Mademoiselle Miss": Letters from an American Girl*

Serving with the Rank of Lieutenant in a French Army Hospital at the Front, preface by Richard C. Cabot (Boston: Butterfield, 1916), 76–77.

34. For an examination of these values and how they gained expression in American medicine in the nineteenth and twentieth centuries, extending through "general practice" of the 1950s and '60s, see Paul E. Stepansky, *In the Hands of Doctors: Touch and Trust in Medical Care* (Santa Barbara: Praeger, 2016).

35. "The flu is back again and everybody has it, including me. I've run a temperature of one hundred and two for three days, can hardly breathe, and have to sleep on four pillows at night." Boylston, *Diary* (ftnt 18), 47.

36. Marjorie Barron Norris, *Sister Heroines: The Roseate Glow of Wartime Nursing, 1914–1918* (Calgary, Alberta, CA: Bunker to Bunker, 2002), 71–72, 79.

37. Boylston, *Diary* (ftnt 19), 91.

38. Essig, *My Trip with Uncle Sam* (ftnt 1), entry of March 23, 1918; Diary of Alice Isaacson, Library and Archives Canada, entry of July 17, 1917 (http://www.bac-lac. gc.ca/eng/discover/military-heritage/first-world-war/canada-nursing-sisters/Pages/item.aspx?PageID=416).

39. E.g., Luard, *Letters* (ftnt 8), 88: "Sister D, the Mother of all the Abdominals, has her marching orders and goes down to Rouen to a General Hospital tomorrow. Her loss is irreparable." Edith Appleton recounts taking care of three sick nurses and a sick VAD at one time: "I have begun to feel like a perpetual night nurse to the sick sisters as I have another one to look after tonight with an abscess in her ear"(*Diaries* [ftnt 20], 123). Maude Essig contracted erysipelas, rediagnosed as "furunculosis [boils] of the nose" in April 1918. Whatever the diagnosis, the condition left the left side of her face swollen and her left eye sealed shut. As late as the following fall, she reported feeling "awfully sick" and relied on "quinine and aspirin in large doses" to keep going (*My Trip with Uncle Sam* [ftnt 1], entries of April 9, April 14, and October 27, 1918). Deaths of nurses are reported by the Canadian nurse Alice Isaacson, *Diary* (ftnt 38), entries of May 5, 1917 and June 6, 1917. Cf. Norris, *Sister Heroines* (ftnt 36), 28, 78, 79.

40. Drew Gilpin Faust, *This Republic of Suffering: Death and The American Civil War* (New York: Vintage, 2008), chapter 1.

41. Ruth G. Haskell, *Helmets and Lipstick: An Army Nurse in World War II* (New York: Putnam's, 1944), 174–175.

42. June Wandrey, *Bedpan Commando: The Story of a Combat Nurse during World War II* (Holland, OH: Elmore), locs 89, 107.

43. Essig, *My Trip with Uncle Sam* (ftnt 1), entry of November 5, 1918, 47.

44. This paragraph draws on the interview material gathered in Diane Burke Fessler, *No Time for Fear: Voices of American Military Nurses in World War II* (East Lansing: Michigan State University Press, 1996), 29–78; Ellen Green Dellane is quoted at 61.

45. Haskell, *Helmets and Lipstick* (ftnt 41), 175.

46. During the war in Vietnam a half century later, cultural and gender sensibilities took another linguistic turn. Among American military nurses, wounded combat soldiers, who now averaged 19, were less "boys" than "kids" or "fellas." A nurse familiarly referred to the men on her ward as "her guys." See, for example, the reminiscences gathered in Patricia Rushton, ed., *Vietnam War Nurses: Personal Accounts of 18 Americans* (Jefferson, NC: McFarland, 2013, 7–8, 44, 67, 110, 112). "They were all young," one remarked, "and they look like your kid brother" (136).

47. Faust, *Republic of Suffering* (ftnt 40), 178, 187.

48. Mary Borden, *The Forbidden Zone* (London: Hesperus, 2008 [1928]); Ellen N. La Motte, *The Backwash of War: The Human Wreckage of the Battlefield as Witnessed by an American Hospital Nurse* (New York: Putnam's, 1916).

49. Isabel Hampton Robb, *Nursing: Its Principles and Practice, for Hospital and*

Private Use (Phila: Saunders, 1893), 67; Isabel Hampton Robb, *Nursing Ethics* (Cleveland: Koeckert, 1900), 34, 40.

50. Harriet Eaton, diary entry of February 14, 1863, quoted in Jane E. Schultz, *Women at the Front: Hospital Workers in Civil War America* (Chapel Hill: University of North Carolina Press, 2004), 123, 287n55.

51. Derr, *"Mademoiselle Miss"* (ftnt 33), 34, 43, 46, 69.

52. Louisa May Alcott, *Life, Letters and Journals*, ed. E. D. Cheney (Boston: Little, Brown, 1928), 118; Derr, *"Mademoiselle Miss"* (ftnt 33), 31.

53. Hannah Ropes, *Civil War Nurse: The Diary and Letters of Hannah Ropes*, ed. John R. Brumgard (Knoxville: University of Tennessee Press, 1980), letter of October 11, 1862, 74; cf. letter of November 5, 1862, 89.

54. Julia A. Houghton Chase, *Mary A. Bickerdyke, "Mother": The Life Story of One who, as Wife, Mother, Army Nurse, Pension Agent and City Missionary, has Touched the Heights and Depths of Human Life* (Lawrence, KS: Journal Publishing House, 1896), 21–22.

55. Sarah Broom Macnaughtan, *A Woman's Diary of the War: Life of a Nurse at the Front* (s.l. Endeavour Compass, 2015 [1915]), 92.

56. Leon Goldman & Glenn E. Cullen, "Some Medical Aspects of Chemical Warfare Agents," *JAMA*, 114:2200–2204, 1940.

57. Editorial, "War Gas Poisoning," *BMJ*, 2:138–139, 1918.

58. Editorial, "Gas in Warfare," *Boston Med. Surg. J.*, 192:1024–1025, 1925; J. A. Ryle, "Discussion on Gas Poisoning," *Proc. R. Soc. Med.*, 13 (war section):47–48, 1920.

59. De Haven Hinkson, "Medical Aspect of Gas Warfare," *J. Natl. Med. Assn.*, 12:1–6, 1920, at p. 5.

60. Stimson, *Letters* (ftnt 8), 80–81.

61. Brittain, *Testament of Youth* (ftnt 9), 360.

62. Quoted in Mary Sarnecky, *A History of the U.S. Army Nurse Corps* (Philadelphia: University of Pennsylvania Press, 1999), 96.

Chapter 5

1. Mary Stollard, quoted in Lyn MacDonald, *The Roses of No Man's Land* (London: Penguin, 1993 [1980]), 232.

2. On the historically contingent nature of the mental disorders caused by war, see especially Edgar Jones & Simon Wessely, "War Syndromes: The Impact of Culture on Medically Unexplained Symptoms," *Med. Hist.*, 49:55–78, 2005 and Edgar Jones, "Historical Approaches to Post-Combat Disorders," *Phil. Trans. R. Soc. B*, 361:533–542, 2006.

3. George Rosen, "Nostalgia: A 'Forgotten' Psychological Disorder," *Psychol. Med.*, 5:340–354, 1975, at 341.

4. Jones, "Historical Approaches to Post-Combat Disorders" (ftnt 2), 536.

5. Annessa C. Stagner, "Healing the Soldier, Restoring the Nation: Representations of Shell Shock in the USA During and After the First World War," *J. Contemp. Hist.*, 49:255–274, 2014.

6. Ben Shephard, *A War of Nerves: Soldiers and Psychiatrists in the Twentieth Century* (Cambridge: Harvard University Press, 2001), 41. Shephard's estimate (409n7) relies on W. Johnson & R. G. Rows, "Neurasthenia and War Neuroses," in *History of the Great War Based on Official Documents: Diseases of War*, vol. 2 (London, 1923), 8–9.

7. Charles S. Meyers, *Shell Shock in France, 1914–1918, Based on a War Diary* (Cambridge: Cambridge University Press, 1940), 13–14.

8. Thomas W. Salmon, *The Care and Treatment of Mental Diseases and War Neuroses ("Shell Shock") in the British Army* (New York: National Committee for Mental Hygiene, 1917), 50, 58.

9. Earl D. Bond, *Thomas W. Salmon—Psychiatrist* (New York: Norton, 1950), 83–84.

10. The shock and residual back pain that followed railway accidents, termed "railway spine," helped legitimize the

concept of functional (i.e., nonanatomi-cal) nervous disorder in the late nine-teenth century. For the railroad compa-nies the notion of functional disorder was a valuable tool in resolving conflicts over responsibility for train accidents. In the Great War, the concept of functional disorder played an analogous role in re-solving issues over the state's responsi-bility for the disabilities of traumatized soldiers. On railway spine in the late nineteenth century, see Ralph Harring-ton, "On the Tracks of Trauma: Railway Spine Reconsidered," *Soc. History. Med.*, 16:209–223, 2003. Edward Brown ex-plores the relationship between railway spine and shell shock in "Between Cow-ardice and Insanity: Shell Shock and the Legitimation of the Neuroses in Great Britain," in: Everett Mendelsohn et al., eds., *Science, Technology and The Mili-tary* (Dordrecht: Kluwer, 1989), 323–345.

11. Julia C. Stimson, *Finding Them-selves: The Letters of an American Army Chief Nurse in a British Hospital in France* (New York: Macmillan, 1918), 41; Dorothea Crewdson, *Dorothea's War: A First World War Nurse Tells her Story*, ed. Richard Crewdson (London: Weidenfeld & Nicolson, 2013), 243; Grace Bagnold, in MacDonald, *Roses of No Man's Land* (ftnt 1), 233.

12. Claire Elise Tisdall, in MacDonald, *Roses of No Man's Land* (ftnt 1), 233–234.

13. Stimson, *Letters* (ftnt 11), letter of June 17, 1917, 41; Amy H. Trench, "Letter to the Members of the American Nurses' Association," *Amer. J. Nurs.*, 12:1179–1180, 1918, quoted at 1179; Crewdson, *Dorothea's War* (ftnt 11), 43; Edith Ap-pleton, *A Nurse at the Front: The First World War Diaries*, ed. R. Cowen (Lon-don: Simon & Schuster UK, 2012), 184. See also Mary Stollard, in MacDonald, *Roses of No Man's Land* (ftnt 1), 231–32.

14. Crewdson, *Dorothea's War* (ftnt 11), 232.

15. *Ibid.*, 236–237.

16. Sophie Hoerner, letter of July 4, 1915, Library & Archives, Canada (http://www.bac-lac.gc.ca/eng/discover/mili-tary-heritage/first-world-war/canada-nursing-sisters/Pages/sophie-hoerner.aspx).

17. Shirley Millard, *I Saw Them Die: Diary and Recollections* ed. Adele Co-mandini (New York: Harcourt Brace, 1936), entry of November 8, 1917, 108–109.

18. See, for example, C. Stanford Read, *Military Psychiatry in Peace and War* (London: Lewis, 1920), 26–27, 30, 89, 141. Read did his best to apply psy-choanalytic principles to his work with psychiatrically impaired soldiers at "D" Block of the Royal Victorian Hospital, Netley.

19. Kate Wilson-Simmie, *Lights Out! The Memoir of Nursing Sister Kate Wil-son, Canadian Army Medical Corps, 1915–1917* (Ottawa: CEF Books, 1981), 133.

20. *Ibid.*, 147.

21. Ella Mae Bongard, *Nobody Ever Wins a War: The World War I Diaries of Ella Mae Bongard, R.N.*, ed. Eric Scott (Ottawa: Janeric Enterprises, 1997), 35.

22. Nelle Fairchild Hefty Rote, *Nurse Helen Fairchild: WWI 1917–1918* (Lewis-burg, PA: privately printed, 2004), 114.

23. Appleton, *Diaries* (ftnt 13), 184.

24. Vera Brittain, *Testament of Youth: An Autobiographical Study of the Years 1900–1925* (London: Penguin, 2015 [1933]), 130.

25. Helen Zenna Smith, *Not so Quiet ... Stepdaughters of War* (New York: Feminist Press of CUNY: 1989 [1930]), 91.

26. Helen Dore Boylston, *Sister: The War Diary of a Nurse* (New York: Ives Washburn, 1927), 69.

27. Freud's and Abraham's remarks, which were made in their respective pre-sentations at the International Psycho-Analytic Congress at Budapest in Sep-tember 1918, were gathered into the vol-ume *Psycho-Analysis and the War Neu-roses* (1909). They are cited in Paul E. Stepansky, *Freud, Surgery, and the Sur-*

geons (New York: Routledge, 1999), 106, 115.

28. Edith Ambrose to Clara D. Noyes, letter of April 9, 1918, American Red Cross Nurse Files, Group 2, 1917–1934. Ambrose was relentless in pursuing appointment to a shell shock facility. On 13 April she again wrote Noyes, advising her of plans to go to Toronto to look into work on shell shock being done by the Canadians, and then back to Boston to learn what she could from a psychologist with "a wonderful filing system." In a third letter to Noyes of 10 May she referred to herself as a specialist, adding, "There are few with my experience in my special line and I feel I would be more valuable to the Red Cross and the War Department, if used in the social service field."

29. Christine Hallett, *Containing Trauma: Nursing Work in the First World War* (Manchester: Manchester University Press, 2009), 163.

30. *Ibid.*, 165, 177.

31. A. D. Macleod, "Shell Shock, Gordon Homes and the Great War," *J. Royal Soc. Med.*, 97:86–89, 2004.

32. Hallett, *Containing Trauma* (ftnt 29), 172–173.

33. Stimson, *Letters* (ftnt 11), 163.

34. Wilson-Simmie, *Lights Out!* (ftnt 19), 133.

35. Lewis R. Yealland, *Hysterical Disorders of Warfare* (London: Macmillan, 1918).

36. Ernest Falzeder & Eva Brabant, eds., *The Correspondence of Sigmund Freud and Sandor Ferenczi, volume 2, 1914–1919* (Cambridge: Harvard University Press, 1996), 264. On the marginal role of psychoanalysis in military psychiatry during WWI, see Stepansky, *Freud, Surgery, and the Surgeons* (ftnt 27), 97–116.

37. E. D. Adrian & L. R. Yealland, "The Treatment of Some Common War Neuroses," *Lancet*, 189:867–872, 1917, at 869.

38. Crewdson, *Dorothea's War* (ftnt 11), 243; Stollard, in MacDonald, *Roses of No Man's Land* (ftnt 1), 232.

39. E.g., Crewdson, *Dorothea's War* (ftnt 11), 273–275; Mary Borden, *The Forbidden Zone* (London: Hesperus, 2008 [1929]), 103. On the military's unwillingness to diagnose women as shell shocked, see Hannah Groch-Begley, "The Forgotten Female Shell-Shock Victims of World War I," *The Atlantic*, September 8, 2014. (https://www.theatlantic.com/health/archive/2014/09/world-war-ones-forgotten-female-shell-shock-victims/378995).

40. Borden, *Forbidden Zone* (ftnt 39), 103.

41. Ellen N. La Motte, *The Backwash of War: The Human Wreckage of the Battlefield as Witnessed by an American Hospital Nurse* (New York: Putnam's, 1916), 239.

42. Henry Viets, "Shell-Shock: A Digest of the English Literature," *JAMA*, 19:1779–1786, 1917, at 1785.

43. Brittain, *Testament of Youth* (ftnt 24), 454.

44. Kate Luard, *Unknown Warriors: The Letters of Kate Luard, RRC and Bar, Nursing Sister in France 1914–1918*, ed. John & Caroline Stevens (Stroud: History Press, 2014), 50.

45. David Forsyth, "Functional Nerve Disease and the Shock of Battle," *Lancet*, 185:1399–1403, 1915, at 1403.

46. Beth Linker, *War's Waste: Rehabilitation in World War I America* (Chicago: University of Chicago Press, 2011), 98ff.

47. *Ibid.*, 142–143. Indeed, the thrust of the postwar rehabilitation movement was to "deveteranize" disabled veterans, i.e., "to transform veterans (as a class) into a group of civilians who would rise and fall by their own merits." That is, they were urged to put their war experience behind them and rejoin the economic mainstream—as if such reintegration were a quick and simple matter. See John Kinder, *Paying with Their Bodies: American War and the Problem of the Disabled Veteran* (Chicago: University of Chicago Press, 2015), 197.

48. Henry Pinsker, et al., *Dynamic*

Supportive Psychotherapy: Handbook of Short-Term Dynamic Psychotherapy (New York: Basic Books, 1991), chap. 1.

49. Appleton, *Diaries* (ftnt 13), 184.

50. Clare Gass, *The War Diary of Clare Gass, 1915–1918*, ed. Susan Mann (Montreal: McGill-Queen's University Press, 2000), entry of June 19, 1915, 32.

51. Millard, *I Saw Them Die* (ftnt 17), entry of 3 April 1918, 21.

52. The notion that shell shock entailed microscopic brain lesions continued to be held by some physicians throughout the war. Among them was the British pathologist Frederick Mott, who treated victims at The Maudsley Hospital in London. He based this claim on postmortem examination of the brains of several British soldiers who, in his view, had died from shell shock. Their brains, according to Mott, resembled the brains of victims of industrial gas poisoning. Both brains provided evidence of extensive capillary hemorrhage. Of course even if Mott were correct, his colleagues countered, brain hemorrhage could only be an "exceptional cause" of shell shock, irrelevant to the overwhelming majority of soldiers "who returned from the front with symptoms of a neurosis." See Viets, "Shell-Shock," (ftnt 42), 1783–1784.

53. Luard, *Letters* (ftnt 44), 167–168; [Kate Norman Derr], "*Mademoiselle Miss*": Letters from an American Girl Serving with the Rank of Lieutenant in a French Army Hospital at the Front, preface by Richard C. Cabot (Boston: Butterfield, 1916), 33.

54. N.A., *A War Nurse's Diary: Sketches from a Belgian Hospital* (New York: Macmillan, 1918), 90.

55. Appleton, *Diaries* (ftnt 13), 184.

56. Agnes Warner, *'My Beloved Poilus'* (St. John: Barnes, 1917), 11.

57. Gass, *War Diary* (ftnt 50), 32.

58. Sarah Macnaughtan, *A Woman's Diary of the War: Life of a Nurse at the Front* (South Yorkshire: Pen & Sword, 2015 [1915]), 92.

59. Beatrice Hopkinson, *Nursing Through Shot & Shell: A Great War Nurse's Story*, ed. Vivien Newman (South Yorkshire: Pen & Sword, 2014), 67.

60. See Ann Jones, *They Were Soldiers: How the Wounded Return from America's Wars—The Untold Story* (Chicago: Haymarket, 2013), chapter 1.

61. Luard, *Letters* (ftnt 44), 166; Derr, "*Mademoiselle Miss*" (ftnt 53), 21.

62. On Kohut's theory of self development, which emerged in the 1970s and '80s as an alternative to Freud's theory of instinctual development, see his final work, *How Does Analysis Cure?*, edited by Arnold Goldberg with the collaboration of Paul E. Stepansky (Chicago: University of Chicago Press, 1984).

63. Crewdson, *Dorothea's War* (ftnt 11), 273–275.

Chapter 6

1. Helen Dore Boylston, *Sister: The War Diary of a Nurse* (New York: Ives Washburn, 1927), entry of 24 October 1918, 89.

2. There is abundant secondary literature on the Great Pandemic of 1918. Excellent, readable overviews are provided by Alfred W. Crosby's two books, *Epidemic and Peace, 1918* (Westport, CT: Greenwood, 1976) and *America's Forgotten Pandemic: The Influenza of 1918*, 2nd ed. (Cambridge: Cambridge University Press, 2003 [1989]); John M. Barry, *The Great Influenza: The Epic Story of the Deadliest Plague in History* (New York: Viking, 2004); and Nancy K. Bristow, *American Pandemic: The Lost Worlds of the 1918 Influenza Epidemic* (Oxford: Oxford University Press, 2012). Those interested in the pandemic's impact on the American Expeditionary Force and the war in general should turn to Carol R. Byerly, *Fever of War: The Influenza Epidemic in the U.S. Army during World War I* (New York: New York University Press, 2005). A lively account of the search for the virus that caused the pandemic in the decades after the war is Gina Kolata, *Flu: The Story of the Great Influenza Pandemic of 1918 and the*

Search for the Virus That Caused It (New York: Farrar, Straus and Giroux, 2011).

3. On the outbreak of flu in Philadelphia following the Liberty Loan Parade of September 28, with an abundance of striking statistics, see especially Crosby, *Epidemic and Peace* (ftnt 2), 70–90.

4. Jennifer D. Keene, *World War I: The American Soldier Experience* (Lincoln: University of Nebraska Press, 2011 [2006]), 128–129; Barry, *Great Influenza* (ftnt 2), 304–306.

5. Cited in Byerly, *Fever of War* (ftnt 2), 6; Keene, *World War I* (ftnt 4), 167.

6. Lavinia L. Dock, et al., *History of the American Red Cross* (New York: Macmillan, 1922), 404–410.

7. Thomas D. Brock, *Robert Koch: A Life in Medicine and Bacteriology* (Washington, D.C.: ASM Press, 1998 [1988]), 14–16.

8. Regina Morantz-Sanchez, *Sympathy and Science: Women Physicians in American Medicine* (Chapel Hill: University of North Carolina Press, 1985), 235–236; Jonathan Liebenau, *Medical Science and Medical Industry: The Formation of the American Pharmaceutical Industry* (Baltimore: Johns Hopkins, 1987), 50–51.

9. Brock, *Robert Koch* (ftnt 7), 278–285.

10. John F. Brundage & G. Dennis Shanks, "Deaths from Bacterial Pneumonia During 1918–19 Influenza Pandemic," *Emerging Infectious Diseases*, 14:1193–1199, 2008; David M. Morens, Jeffery K. Taubenberger & Anthony S. Fauci, "Role of Bacterial Pneumonia as a Cause of Death in Pandemic Influenza: Implications for Pandemic Influenza Preparedness," *Journal of Infectious Diseases*, 198:962–970, 2008.

11. Edith Appleton, *A Nurse at the Front: The First World War Diaries of Sister Edith Appleton*, ed. Ruth Cowen (London: Simon & Schuster, 2012), 220.

12. Nancy O'Brien Wagner, ed., *Alice in France: The World War I Letters of Alice M. O'Brien* (St. Paul, MN: Minnesota Historical Society Press, 2017), loc 1948.

13. Brook B. Cameron & Janice C. Collins, eds., *Finding Helen: The Letters, Photographs and Diary of a WWI Battlefield Nurse*, 2nd ed. (s.l.: s.n., 2014.), 213; Nora Saltonstall, *The World War I Letters of Nora Saltonstall*, ed. Judith S. Graham (Boston: Northeastern Univ. Press, 2004), 196, 198.

14. Boylston, *Diary* (ftnt 1), 121.

15. Shirley Millard, *I Saw Them Die: Diary and Recollections*, ed. Adele Comandini (New York: Harcourt, Brace, 1936), 18–19; Alma S. Woolley, "A Hoosier Nurse in France: The World War I Diary of Maude Frances Essig (https://scholarworks.iu.edu/journals/index.php/imh/article/view/10683/15077), entry of October 7, 1918; Mary Dobson, letter of September 28, 1918, in Lynn MacDonald, *The Roses of No Man's Land* (London: Penguin, 1993), 322.

16. Dorothy Deming, "Influenza—1918: Reliving the Great Epidemic," *Am. J. Nurs.*, 57:1308–1309, 1957, at 1309.

17. Beatrice Hopkinson, *Nursing through Shot & Shell: A Great War Nurse's Story*, ed. Vivien Newman (South Yorkshire: Pen & Sword, 2014), 96–97. On the failure of bacterial serums, see *Diary of Alice Isaacson*, Library and Archives Canada (http://www.bac-lac.gc.ca/eng/discover/military-heritage/first-world-war/canada-nursing-sisters/Pages/alice-isaacson.aspx), entry of October 31, 1918.

18. Kate Cumming, *The Journal of a Confederate Nurse*, ed. Richard Barksdale Harwell (Baton Rouge: Louisiana State University Press, 1959 [1866]), entry of 3 November 1863, 166.

19. Sarah Smith Sampson, July 1862, quoted in Libby MacCaskill & David Novak, *Ladies on the Field: Two Civil War Nurses from Maine on the Battlefields of Virginia* (Livermore, ME: Signal Tree, 1996), 60.

20. Kitty Kenyon (VAD at General Hospital No. 4, Camiers) and Sister Henrietta Beanland (St. Luke's War Hospital, Bradford), in Macdonald, *Roses of No Man's Land* (ftnt 15), 318–319, 320–321.

21. Henrietta Beanland (op cit.), Ali-

son Strathy (American Red Cross Aide, French Field Hospital), Lloyd, Gwynnedd Lloyd (VAD, University War Hospital, Southampton), in Macdonald, *Roses of No Man's Land* (ftnt 15), 321–323.

22. Elizabeth Cobbs, *The Hello Girls: America's First Women Soldiers* (Cambridge: Harvard University Press, 2017), 134.

23. Appleton, *Diaries* (ftnt 11), 102; Essig, "World War I Diary" (ftnt 15, entry of October 27, 1918; Boylston, *Diary* (ftnt 1), entry of 6 November 1918, 91.

24. Dorothea Crewdson, *Dorothea's War: A First World War Nurse Tells her Story*, ed. Richard Crewdson (London: Weidenfeld & Nicolson, 2013), 300, 303.

25. Many students serving on infected wards contracted influenza themselves and at least 10 died. Anna C. Jamme, "The Army School of Nursing," *Amer. J. Nurs.*, 19:179–184, 1918.

26. Deming, "Influenza—1918" (ftnt 16); quoted in Bristow, *American Pandemic* (ftnt 2), 134.

27. Susan Zeiger, *In Uncle Sam's Service: Women Workers with the American Expeditionary Force, 1917–1919* (Ithaca: Cornell University Press, 1999), 132.

28. Vera Brittain, *Testament of Youth: An Autobiographical Study of the Years 1900–1925*, intro. Mark Bostridge (London: Penguin, 2015 [1933]), 185, 187.

29. Grace Anderson, *Pride of America: The Letters of Grace Anderson, U.S. Army Nurse Corps, World War I*, ed. Shari Lynn Wigle (Rockville, MD: Seaboard Press, 2007), 113; Katharine Wilson-Simmie, *Lights Out! The Memoir of Nursing Sister Kate Wilson, Canadian Army Medical Corps 1915–1917* (Ottawa: CEF, 2004), 177–187.

30. "The Journal of Emma Elizabeth Weaver," in *Nurses of World War One: Service beyond Expectations*, ed., Lorraine Luciano & Casandra Jewell (Carlisle, PA: Army Heritage Center Foundation, 2006), 208 (p. 51 of original journal).

31. *Ibid.*, 226 (p. 80 of original journal).

32. *Ibid.*, 229 (p. 82 of original journal).

33. On the role of American women physicians in World War I and its aftermath, see Ellen S. More, "'A Certain Restless Ambition': Women Physicians and World War I," *Amer. Quart.*, 41:1989, 636–660; Lettie Gavin, *American Women in World War I* (Niwot, CO: University Press of Colorado, 1997), 157–178; Kimberly Jensen, *Mobilizing Minerva: American Women in the First World War* (Urbana: University of Illinois Press, 2008), 77–97, 103–115; and Judith Bellafaire & Mercedes Herrera Graf, *Women Doctors in War* (College Station: Texas A&M University Press, 2009), 21–31. Statistics on AWH No. 1's service while based in Luzancy are in Jensen, *Mobilizing Minerva*, 110.

34. E.M.W., "Letters from Nurses in Service," *Amer. J. Nurs.*, 69:715–718, 1919.

35. Cumming, *Journal* (ftnt 18), entry of 12 April 1862, 16: "Other ladies have their special patients, whom they never leave. One of them, from Natchez, Miss., has been constantly by a young man, badly wounded, ever since she came here, and the doctors say that she has been the means of saving his life."

36. Saltonstall, *Letters* (ftnt 13), 179–180.

37. Keene, *World War I* (ftnt 4), 166.

38. AEF nurse Nellie Dingley, herself a casualty of the flu, quoted in Gavin, *American Women in World War I* (ftnt 33), 63.

39. See, e.g., Cumming, *Journal* (ftnt 18), 32–33, 73, 103, 182; Louisa May Alcott, *Hospital Sketches* (Mineola, NY: Dover, 2006 [1863]), 34; Amanda Akin Sterns, *The Lady Nurse of Ward E* (New York: Baker & Taylor, 1909), 126.

40. Jean V. Berlin, ed., *A Confederate Nurse: The Diary of Ada W. Bacot, 1860–1863* (Columbia, SC: University South Carolina Press, 1994), 141.

41. [Kate Norman Derr], *"Mademoiselle Miss": Letters from an American Girl Serving with the Rank of Lieutenant in a French Army Hospital at the Front*, pre-

face by R. C. Cabot (Boston: Butterfield, 1916), 21.

42. Michael C. C. Adams, *Living Hell: The Dark Side of the Civil War* (Baltimore: Johns Hopkins University Press, 2014), 23–24.

43. Nicholas Senn, *Medico-Surgical Aspects of the Spanish-American War* (Chicago: American Medical Association Press, 1900), 171–172.

44. Vincent J. Cirillo, *Bullets and Bacilli: The Spanish-American War and Military Medicine* (New Brunswick, Rutgers University Press, 2004), 92ff.

45. *Ibid.*, 87.

46. Nurses Helen B. Schuler, Florence M. Kelly, and Margaret A. Shanks, quoted in Mercedes H. Graf, "Women Nurses in the Spanish-American War," *Minerva*, 19:3–19, 2001, at 8–9.

47. Boylston, *Diary* (ftnt 1), entry of October 24, 1918, 89; Hopkinson, *Nursing through Shot & Shell* (ftnt 17), ebook loc 122.

48. Sheila Goostray, "Mary Adelaide Nutting," *Amer. J. Nurs.*, 58:1524–1529, 1958, at 1527.

49. Darlene Clark Hine, *Black Women in White: Racial Conflict and Cooperation in the Nursing Profession, 1890–1950* (Bloomington: Indiana University Press, 1989), 94–95.

50. Bacot's diaries record only a single instance of sustained bodily nursing care, and that involved not a soldier but Dr. James McIntosh, a young surgeon whom she befriended. When McIntosh developed erysipelas [a deep skin infection] in February 1862, Bacot, solicitous and maternal, washed his hands and face, combed his hair, and "bathed his head & rubbed his temples until he slept," noting all the while that this arrangement was out of the ordinary for both of them: "He has permitted me to nurse him a good deal, & realy [*sic*] seems to like me to wait on him" Berlin, *Confederate Nurse* (ftnt 40), 83–89. Cornelia Hancock's remark is from a letter to her mother of May 1864, in Cornelia Hancock, *Letters of a Civil War Nurse: Cornelia Hancock,*

1863–1865, ed. Henrietta Jacquette (Lincoln: University of Nebraska Press, 1998), 86.

51. Bellafaire & Graf, *Women Doctors in War* (ftnt 33), 26–27.

52. This section relies on Thomas Kuhn's theory of paradigms in relation to scientific problem-solving and scientific progress, first adumbrated in his seminal work, *The Structure of Scientific Revolutions* (Chicago: University of Chicago Press, 1970) and elaborated in later writings, many collected in *The Essential Tension: Selected Studies in Tradition and Change* (Chicago: University of Chicago Press, 1977). I have used Kuhn's perspective on paradigms, incommensurability, and paradigm change in a previous work, Paul E. Stepansky, *Psychoanalysis at the Margins* (New York: Other Press, 2009), 168–171, 231–233.

53. Victoria A. Harden, *Inventing the NIH: Federal Biomedical Research Policy, 1887–1937* (Baltimore: Johns Hopkins University Press, 1986), 41; Gwyn MacFarlane, *Alexander Fleming: The Man and the Myth* (Cambridge: Harvard University Press, 1984), 54–55.

54. MacFarlane, *Alexander Fleming* (ftnt 53), 84–88.

55. Wagner, *Alice in France* (ftnt 11), loc 1940.

56. *Diary of Alice Isaacson* (ftnt 17), entry of October 31, 1918.

57. Arlene W. Keeling, "'Alert to the Necessities of the Emergency': U.S. Nursing During the 1918 Influenza Pandemic," *Public Health Reports*, 125(suppl. 3):105–112, 2010; cited at 110.

58. Cameron & Collins, *Finding Helen* [ftnt 13], 230. Cf. 232: "We are pretty tough guys living in tents."

59. Woolley, "A Hoosier Nurse in France" (ftnt 15), entry of September 30, 1918; Wagner, *Alice in France* (ftnt 11), entry of May 3, 1918; N.A. (possibly M. E. Clark), *A War Nurse's Diary: Sketches from a Belgian Field Hospital* (New York: Macmillan, 1918), 67.

60. Millard, *I Saw Them Die* (ftnt 15), 19.

61. I use the phrase "nursing through" as analogous to the psychoanalytic concept of "working through," the repetitive reexperiencing and re-visioning of painful intrapsychic conflicts from the past.

62. Boylston, *Diary* (ftnt 1), entry of May 19, 1918, 56.

63. "Banality of catastrophe" is a play on the subtitle of Hannah Arendt's powerful and still unsettling study, *Eichmann in Jerusalem: A Report on the Banality of Evil* (New York: Viking, 1963).

64. G. Dennis Shanks, et al., "Low but Highly Variable Mortality among Nurses and Physicians during the Influenza Pandemic of 1918–1919," *Influenza and Other Respiratory Viruses*, 5:213–219, 2011.

Chapter 7

1. Helen Doyle Boylston, *Sister: The War Diary of a Nurse* (New York: Washburn, 1927), entry one year after the Armistice, 105.

2. The history of the American nurse practitioner movement is ably charted by Julie Fairman in *Making Room in the Clinic: Nurse Practitioners and the Evolution of Modern Health Care* (New Brunswick: Rutgers University Press, 2008). My own perspective on nurse practitioners, which differs from Fairman's in certain respects, is in Paul E. Stepansky, *In the Hands of Doctors: Touch and Trust in Medical Care* (Santa Barbara: Praeger, 2016; exp. pbk. ed., Keynote Books, 2017), ch. 11 ("What Do Nurse Practitioners Practice?").

3. The pledge was written by Lystra E. Gretter and a Committee for the Farrand Training School for Nurses in Detroit. See Alice Tarbell Crathern, *In Detroit Courage was the Fashion: The Contribution of Women to the Development of Detroit from 1701 to 1951* (Detroit: Wayne State University Press, 1953), 80–81. The last sentence of the pledge reads: "With loyalty will I endeavor to aid the physician, in his work,

and devote myself to the welfare of those committed to my care." The pledge of 1893 was revised in 1935, at which time the reference to "the physician" in characterizing nurses' obligation was retained.

4. Susan M. Reverby, *Ordered to Care: The Dilemma of American Nursing, 1850–1945* (Cambridge: Cambridge University Press, 1987), 123–124; Patricia D'Antonio, *American Nursing: A History of Knowledge, Authority, and the Meaning of Work* (Baltimore: John Hopkins University Press, 2010), 135.

5. LaVonne Telshaw Camp, *Lingering Fever: A World War II Nurse's Memoir* (Jefferson, NC: McFarland, 1997), 170.

6. Lynn Calmes Kohut, in Patricia Rushton, ed., *Vietnam War Nurses: Personal Accounts of 18 Americans* (Jefferson, NC: McFarland, 2013), 126. By the late '60s, nurses serving in Vietnam were starting and monitoring IVs as part of their daily routine (Lou Ellen Bell, *Ibid.*, 29).

7. Susan C. McCall, "Lessons Learned by Army Nurses in Combat: A Historical Review," Individual Study Project (unclassified), 15 April 1993, Army War College, Carlisle Barracks, PA. Mary Lou Ostergren-Bruner, a Vietnam nurse with OR training, recalls practicing triage on the injured in a tent hospital set up at Sam Houston Naval Hospital by, among other things, "traching a goat." See Rushton, *Vietnam War Nurses* (ftnt 6), 135.

8. Bernadette J. Harrod, *Fort Chastity, Vietnam, 1969: A Nurse's Story of the Vietnam War* (s.l.: iUniverse, 2015), loc. 332.

9. Elizabeth Scannell-Desch & Mary Ellen Doherty, eds., *Nurses in War: Voices from Iraq and Afghanistan* (New York: Springer Publishing, 2012), 194–195. For these contemporary nurses, the need to perform such procedures represented desirable learning opportunities that added to their clinical skill set (e.g., 34, 192).

10. On these interwar developments,

see D'Antonio, *American Nursing* (ftnt 4), 123; Reverby, *Ordered to Care* (ftnt 4), 169–171; and Barbara Brooks Tomblin, *G.I. Nightingales: The Army Nurse Corps in World War II* (Lexington: University of Kentucky Press, 1996), 1–12.

11. D'Antonio, *American Nursing* (ftnt 4), 165.

12. Virginia S. Thatcher, *History of Anesthesia—With Emphasis on the Nurse Specialist* (Phila: Lippincott, 1953), 181ff.

13. McCall, "Lessons Learned" (ftnt 7), 8.

14. The manner in which different aspects of gender and sexuality enter into and fall out of American nursing, civilian and military, over time, is an important but surprisingly neglected topic. Of particular interest would be studies that compared and contrasted the roles of gender and sexuality across the successive armed conflicts in which America has engaged over the course of its brief history. Such research could profitably engage a range of historian sensibilities and specialties, not just those of military and nursing history and gender studies. A noteworthy contribution to this project is Margaret Sandelowski, *Devices and Desires: Gender, Technology, and American Nursing* (Chapel Hill: University of North Carolina Press, 2000). The gendered dimension of military nursing in one of America's wars is thoughtfully examined in Kara Dixon Vuic, *Officer, Nurse, Woman: The Army Nurse Corps in the Vietnam War* (Baltimore: Johns Hopkins University Press, 2011).

15. Florence Nightingale, *Notes on Nursing: What It Is and What It Is Not* (New York: Appleton, 1860 [1859]), 126–130.

16. I. H. Robb, *Nursing Ethics* (Cleveland: Koeckert, 1900), 34, 40.

17. Official Film, War Department, Misc. 1173, "Army Nurse," produced by Army Pictorial Service, Signal Corps, publication date 1945. The film is viewable at: https://www.youtube.com/watch?v=da5MVQKi7Rc&t=217s).

18. Slowing down the rate of drip, the researchers found, was the way to eliminate what they termed as "speed shock." See Harold Thomas Hyman & Samuel Hirshfeld, "Studies of Velocity and the Response to Intravenous Injections: III. Technic of the Intravenous Drip in Clinical Practice," *JAMA*, 96:1221–1223, 1931, and Samuel Hirshfeld, Harold Thomas Hyman, & Justine Wanger, "Influence of Velocity on the Response to Intravenous Injections," *Arch. Intern. Med.*, 47:259–287, 1931. As far back as 1888, Rudolph Matas, while removing a thyroid tumor (thyroidectomy), used intravenous infusions of saline solution to counteract his patient's acute anemia See Isidore Cohn with Hermann B. Deutsch, *Rudolph Matas: A Biography of One of the Great Pioneers in Surgery* (New York: Doubleday, 1960), 222–230.

19. Julia Polchlopek Scott, in Diane Burke Fessler, *No Time for Fear: Voices of American Military Nurses in World War II* (East Lansing: Michigan State University Press, 1995), 58. Cf. Aloha Drenman Sanchez, in Fessler, 117: "Then one of the doctors couldn't get an IV started, and I realized he was drunk, so I pushed him aside and started it myself."

20. Sally Hitchcock Putnam, *Letters Home: Memoirs of one Army Nurse in the Southwest Pacific in World War II* (s.l.: AuthorHouse, 2004), 143–144, 221.

21. Sanchez, in Fessler, *No Time for Fear* (ftnt 19), 116.

22. Tomblin, *G.I. Nightingales* (ftnt 10), 14–15.

23. *Ibid.*, 19, 16.

24. *Ibid.*, 128.

25. Putnam, *Letters Home* (ftnt 20), 97.

26. *Ibid.*, letter of February 8, 1944, 101.

27. *Ibid.*, 206–207.

28. Penny Starns, *Nurses at War, Women on the Frontline, 1939–45* (Gloucestershire: Sutton, 2000), 72.

29. Marlene Hein Burrell, in Fessler, *No Time for Fear* (ftnt 19), 126.

30. Elsie Sours, in Fessler, *No Time for Fear* (ftnt 19), 106–107; Aubrey Lampier,

in Fessler, 34; Camp, *Lingering Fever* (ftnt 5), 16.

31. Putnam, *Letters Home* (ftnt 20), 60.

32. Teresa M. O'Neill, *"I Wanted to Do Something for the Country": Experiences of Military Nurses in World War II,* unpublished doctoral Dissertation, University of Miami, 2003, 121.

33. Putnam, *Letters Home* (ftnt 20), 31, 170.

34. Tomblin, *G.I. Nightingales* (ftnt 10), 20, 25.

35. O'Neill, *"I Wanted to Serve My Country"* (ftnt 32), 121–122.

36. Elsie Ott Mandot, in Fessler, *No Time for Fear* (ftnt 19), 109.

37. Jean Yunker Johnson, in Fessler, *No Time for Fear* (ftnt 19), 112; Tomblin, *G.I. Nightingales* (ftnt 10), 62.

38. *Ibid.*, 129–130.

39. *Medical Department of the United States Army in The World War, Volume II: Administration American Expeditionary Forces,* prepared under the direction of Maj. Gen. M. W. Ireland, by Colonel Joseph H. Ford (Washington, D.C.: U.S. Government Printing Office, 1927), 324–327. The descriptions of activity in the Aubervilliers train stations en route to base hospitals comes from Marie van Horst, *War Letters of an American Woman* (New York: John Lane, 1916), 91–92.

40. Elizabeth Norman, *Women at War: The Story of Fifty Military Nurses Who Served in Vietnam* (Philadelphia: University of Pennsylvania Press, 1990), 35.

41. *Ibid.*, 37–38.

42. *Ibid.*, 38.

43. Katharine Wilson-Simmie, *Lights Out! The Memoir of Nursing Sister Kate Wilson, Canadian Army Medical Corps 1915–1917* (Ottawa: CEF Books, 2004), 163; Norman, *Women at War* (ftnt 40), 42–43.

44. Alma S. Woolley, "A Hoosier Nurse in France: The World War I Diary of Maude Frances Essig" (https://scholarworks.iu.edu/journals/index.php/imh/

article/view/10683/15077), entry of October 4, 1918; Beatrice Hopkinson, *Nursing through Shot & Shell: A Great War Nurse's Story,* ed. Vivien Newman (South Yorkshire: Pen & Sword, 2014), 103; Elizabeth Lewis, "Letters of Elizabeth Lewis," in Lorraine Luciano & Casandra Jewell, eds., *Army Nurses of World War One: Service Beyond Expectations* (Carlisle, PA: Army Heritage Center Foundation, 2006), 74–77.

45. Camp, *Lingering Fever* (ftnt 5), 41. Certainly not all nurses and doctors felt this way. See for example Florence Edgiton, in Fessler, *No Time for Fear* (ftnt 19), 108.

46. Norman, *Women at War* (ftnt 40), 67.

47. Lou Ellen Bell, in Rushton, *Vietnam War Nurses* (ftnt 6), 35.

48. Norman, *Women at War* (ftnt 40), 66–67.

49. *Ibid.*, 65; Linda Caldwell, in Rushton, *Vietnam War Nurses* (ftnt 6), 68.

50. The work of Regina Morantz-Sanchez is especially illuminating of this binary and the major protagonists at the two poles. See Regina Morantz, "Feminism, Professionalism, and Germs: The Thought of Mary Putnam Jacobi and Elizabeth Blackwell," *Amer. Quar.,* 34:459–478, 1982, with a slightly revised version of the paper in Regina Morantz-Sanchez, *Sympathy and Science: Women Physicians in American Medicine* (Chapel Hill: University of North Carolina Press, 2000 [1985]), 184–202.

51. Nicholas Senn, *Medico-Surgical Aspects of the Spanish American War* (Chicago: AMA Press, 1900), 318–319.

52. Juanita Redmond, quoted in Tomblin, *G.I. Nightingales* (ftnt 10), 29.

53. Katherine Volk, *Buddies in Budapest* (Los Angeles: Kellaway-Ide, 1936), 136; Maude Mortimer, *A Green Tent in Flanders* (Garden City: Doubleday, Page, 1918), 83; Kate Luard, *Unknown Warriors: The Letters of Kate Luard, RRC and Bar, Nursing Sister in France, 1914–1918,* ed. John & Caroline Stevens (Stroud: History Press, 2014), 68.

54. Katherine Jump and Anna Mae Hayes are quoted from the Oral History Project, Military History Institute, Carlisle, PA, as cited in McCall, "Lessons Learned by Army Nurses in Combat" (ftnt 7), 16.

55. Mary Lou Ostergren-Bruner, in Rushton, *Vietnam War Nurses* (ftnt 6), 137.

56. Starns, *Nurses at War* (ftnt 28), 73.

57. Elizabeth R. Barker, in Rushton, *Vietnam War Nurses* (ftnt 6), 7–8.

58. Jean V. Berlin, "Introduction," in Jean V. Berlin, ed., *A Confederate Nurse: The Diary of Ada W. Bacot, 1850–1863* (Columbia: University of South Carolina Press, 1994), 11.

59. During Harriet Eaton's visit to the Lincoln Hospital in Washington in October 1864, a soldier called out to her: "oh! Mrs. Eaton, that mustard plaster you put on saved my life, I have the marks of it now, verily it must have been a strong one." Jane E. Schultz, ed., *The Birth Place of Souls: The Civil War Nursing Diary of Harriet Eaton* (New York: Oxford University Press, 2011), 154.

60. Nelle Fairchild Hefty Rote, *Nurse Helen Fairchild: WWI 1917–1918* (Lewisburg, PA: privately printed, 2004), letter of May 1917, 25–26; Emily Elizabeth Parsons, *Memoir* (Boston: Little, Brown, 1880), 80–81,

61. Although individual nurses occasionally invoked Christian faith as a support during their time of troubles, there is little in the World War I diaries, letters, and memoirs consulted in his study that support Jonathan Ebel's thesis, viz., that notions of Christian struggle and righteousness and the assurance, on death, of immediate salvation, helped soldiers accept the horror before them. More typical of the nurses, I believe, is the sentiment of the artist and poet Paul Nash, who wrote to his wife from the Ypres Salient in November 1917: "I have seen the most frightful nightmare of a country more conceived by Dante or Poe than by nature, unspeakable, utterly indescribable...no glimmer of God's hand is seen anywhere...It is unspeakable, godless, hopeless." Quoted in Rote, *Nurse Helen Fairchild* (ftnt 60), 195. Ebel's thesis is set forth in *Faith in the Fight: Religion and the American Soldier in the Great War* (Princeton: Princeton University Press, 2010). Nash conveys plain spoken horror where the nurses tend to more oblique, if caustic asides. "Can God be on our side—everyone is asking—when His (alleged!) Department always intervenes in favor of the enemy at all our best moments." This is Kate Luard during the Third Battle of Ypres on 2 August 1917. See Luard, *Letters* (ftnt 53), 135.

62. Luard, *Letters* (ftnt 53), 90.

Bibliography

Nurses' Diaries, Letters and Memoirs

Archival Sources

Alma A. Clarke Papers, 1914–1946, Special Collections Department, Bryn Mawr College Library, Bryn Mawr, PA. ("Training Notebook of 1914").

American Red Cross Nurse Files, Group 2, 1917–1934 (letters of Edith Ambrose).

Barbara Bates Center for the Study of the History of Nursing, University of Pennsylvania School of Nursing, Philadelphia, PA. (letters of Caroline R. Bauer and Nancy Josephine Klase).

Library & Archives, Canada, "The Call to Duty: Canadian Nursing Sisters" (http://www.bac-lac.gc.ca/eng/discover/military-heritage/first-world-war/canada-nursing-sisters/Pages/canada-nursing-sisters.aspx) (diary of 1917 of Alice Isaacson, letters of Sophie Hoerner).

Maude Essig World War I Diary, Illinois Wesleyan Historical Collections, Illinois Wesleyan University, Bloomington, IL ("My Trip Abroad with Uncle Sam, 1917–1919").

Published Sources

Alcott, Louisa May, *Life, Letters and Journals*, ed. E. D. Cheney. Boston: Little, Brown, 1928.

Anderson, Grace, *Pride of America: The Letters of Grace Anderson, U.S. Army Nurse Corps, World War I*, ed. Shari Lynn Wigle. Rockville, MD: Seaboard, 2007.

Anderson, Isabel, *Zigzagging: An American Female Nurse's Experience during WWI*. Washington, D.C.: Westphalia, 2015.

Appleton, Edith, *A Nurse at the Front: The First World War Diaries*, ed. R. Cowen. London: Simon & Schuster UK, 2012.

Bacot, Ada W., *A Confederate Nurse: The Diary of Ada W. Bacot, 1860–1863*, ed. Jean V. Berlin. Columbia: University of South Carolina Press, 2000.

Bagnold, Enid, *A Diary Without Dates*. London: Heinemann, 1918.

Bongard, Ella Mae, *Nobody Ever Wins A War: The World War I Diaries of Ella Mae Bongard, R.N.*, ed. Eric Scott. Ottawa: Janeric Enterprises, 1997.

Borden, Mary, *The Forbidden Zone*, ed. H. Hutchison. London: Hesperus, 2008 [1928].

Boylston, Helen Dore, *Sister: The War Diary of a Nurse*. n.l.: Kismet, 2018 [1927]).

Brittain, Vera, *Testament of Youth: An Autobiographical Study of the Years 1900–1925*. London: Penguin, 2015 [1933].

Bron, Alice, *Diary of a Nurse in South Africa: Being A Narrative of Experiences in The Boer and English Hospital Service*. London: Chapman & Hall, 1901.

Bucklin, Sophronia, *In Hospital and Camp in the American Civil War* (s.l.: s.n., 2016 [1869]).

Cameron, Brook B., and Collins, Janice C., eds., *Finding Helen: The Letters, Photographs and Diary of a WWI Battlefield Nurse*, 2nd ed. s.l.: s.n., 2014.

Camp, LaVonne Telshaw, *Lingering Fever: A World War II Nurse's Memoir* Jefferson, NC: McFarland, 1997.

"A Canadian Nurse in France," *American Journal of Nursing*, 17:790–791, June 1917.

[Clarke, M. E.], *A War Nurse's Diary: Sketches from a Belgian Field Hospital.* New York: Macmillan, 1918.

Cluett, Frances, *Your Daughter Fanny: War Letters of Frances Cluett, VAD*, ed. Bill Rompkey and Bert Riggs. St. John's NL: Flanker, 2006.

Crewdson, Dorothea, *Dorothea's War: A First World War Nurse Tells Her Story*, ed. Richard Crewdson. London: Weidenfeld & Nicolson, 2013.

Cumming, Kate, *The Journal of a Confederate Nurse*, ed. Richard B. Harwell. Baton Rouge: LSU Press, 1987 [1866].

De Ford, William Harper, *Lectures on General Anaesthetics in Dentistry.* Pittsburgh: Lee S. Smith, 1912.

Dennie, Fannie, "The Experience of an Army Nurse," *Trained Nurse Hospital Review*, 22:111–118, 1899.

Derr, Kate Norman, *"Mademoiselle Miss": Letters from an American Girl Serving with the Rank of Lieutenant in a French Army Hospital at the Front*, preface by Richard C. Cabot. Boston: Butterfield, 1916.

E. M. W., "Letters from Nurses in Service," *American Journal of Nursing*, 69:715–718, 1919.

Eaton, Harriet, *This Birth Place of Souls: The Civil War Nursing Diary of Harriet Eaton*, ed. Jane E. Schultz. New York: Oxford University Press, 2011.

Fessler, Diane Burke, *No Time for Fear: Voices of American Military Nurses in World War II.* East Lansing: Michigan State University Press, 1996.

Gass, Clare, *The War Diary of Clare Gass, 1915–1918*, ed. Susan Mann. Montreal: McGill-Queen's University Press, 2000.

Hancock, Cornelia, *Letters of a Civil War Nurse, 1863–1865*, ed. Henrietta Jaquette. Lincoln: University of Nebraska Press, 1998 [1937].

Harrod, Bernadette J., *Fort Chastity, Vietnam, 1969: A Nurse's Story of the Vietnam War.* s.l.: iUniverse, 2015.

Haskell, Ruth G., *Helmets and Lipstick: An Army Nurse in World War II.* New York: Putnam's, 1944.

Holland, Laura Holland, and Forbes, Mildred, *War-Torn Exchanges: The Lives and Letters of Nursing Sisters Laura Holland and Mildred Forbes*, ed. Andrea McKenzie. Vancouver: UBC Press, 2016.

Holland, Mary Gardner, *Our Army Nurses: Stories from Women in the Civil War.* Roseville, MN: Edinborough, 1998 [1895].

Hopkinson, Beatrice, *Nursing through Shot & Shell: A Great War Nurse's Story*, ed. Vivien Newman. South Yorkshire: Pen & Sword, 2014.

La Motte, Ellen N., *The Backwash of War: The Human Wreckage of the Battlefield as Witnessed by an American Hospital Nurse.* New York: Putnam's, 1916.

Lewis, Elizabeth, "Letters of Elizabeth Lewis," in Lorraine Luciano and Casandra Jewell, eds., *Army Nurses of World War One: Service Beyond Expectations.* Carlisle, PA: Army Heritage Center Foundation, 2006.

Luard, Kate, *Unknown Warriors: The Letters of Kate Luard, RRC and Bar, Nursing Sister in France 1914–1918*, ed. John & Caroline Stevens. Stroud: History Press, 2014.

MacCaskill, Libby, and Novak, David, eds., *Ladies on the Field: Two Civil War Nurses from Maine on the Battlefields of Virginia.* Livermore, ME: Signal Tree, 1996.

MacDonald, Lyn, ed., *The Roses of No Man's Land.* London: Penguin, 1993 [1980].

Macnaughtan, Sarah, *A Woman's Diary of the War: Life of a Nurse at the Front.*

South Yorkshire: Pen & Sword, 2015 [1915].

McDougall, Grace, *A Nurse at the War: Nursing Adventures in Belgium and France*. New York: McBride, 1917.

Millard, Shirley, *I Saw Them Die: Diary and Recollections*. New Orleans, LA: Quid Pro, 2011.

Mortimer, Maude, *A Green Tent in Flanders*. Garden City: Doubleday, Page, 1918.

Norman, Elizabeth, *Women at War: The Story of Fifty Military Nurses Who Served in Vietnam*. Philadelphia: University of Pennsylvania Press, 1990.

Norris, Marjorie Barron, *Sister Heroines: The Roseate Glow of Wartime Nursing, 1914–1918*. Calgary: Bunker to Bunker, 2002.

O'Brien, Alice M., *Alice in France: The World War I Letters of Alice M. O'Brien,* ed. Nancy Wagner. St. Paul, MN: Minnesota Historical Society Press, 2017.

Parsons, Emily Elizabeth, *Memoir: Published for the Benefit of the Cambridge Hospital*. Boston: Little, Brown, 1980.

Putnam, Sally Hitchcock, *Letters Home: Memoirs of One Army Nurse in the Southwest Pacific in World War II*. s.l.: AuthorHouse, 2004.

Ropes, Hannah, *Civil War Nurse: The Diary and Letters of Hannah Ropes,* ed. John R. Brumgard. Knoxville: University of Tennessee Press, 1980.

Rote, Nelle Fairchild Hefty, *Nurse Helen Fairchild: WWI 1917–1918*. Lewisburg, PA: privately printed, 2004.

Rushton, Patricia, ed., *Vietnam War Nurses: Personal Accounts of 18 Americans*. Jefferson, NC: McFarland, 2013.

Saltonstall, Nora, *The World War I Letters of Nora Saltonstall,* ed. Judith S. Graham. Boston: Northeastern University Press, 2004.

Scannell-Desch, Elizabeth, and Doherty, Mary Ellen, eds., *Nurses in War: Voices from Iraq and Afghanistan*. New York: Springer Publishing, 2012.

Sister X, *The Tragedy and Comedy of War Hospitals*. New York: Dutton, 1906.

Stearns, Amanda Akins, *The Lady Nurse of Ward E, 1863–1864*. New York: Baker & Taylor, 1909.

Stimson, Julia C., *Finding Themselves: The Letters of an American Army Chief Nurse in a British Hospital in France*. New York: Macmillan, 1918.

Trench, Amy H., "Letter to the Members of the American Nurses' Association," *American Journal of Nursing,* 12:1179–1180, July 1918.

Van Horst, Marie, *War Letters of an American Woman*. New York: John Lane, 1916.

Wandrey, June, *Bedpan Commando: The Story of a Combat Nurse During World War II*. Holland, OH: Elmore, 1989.

A War Nurse's Diary: Sketches from a Belgian Hospital. New York: Macmillan, 1918.

Warner, Agnes, *'My Beloved Poilus.'* St. John: Barnes, 1917.

Weaver, Emma Elizabeth, *The Journal of Emma Elizabeth Weaver,* ed. Lorraine Luciano and Casandra Jewell. Carlisle, PA: Army Heritage Center Foundation, 2006.

Wilson-Simmie, Katherine, *Lights Out! The Memoir of Nursing Sister Kate Wilson: Canadian Army Medical Corps, 1915–1917*. Ottawa: CEF Books, 2004 [1981].

Wingreen, Amy, "The Poor Men Were So Glad to See Me: A War Nurse in Cuba, 1898," *Missouri Review,* 16:97–130, 1993.

Wolley, Alma S., "Hoosier Nurses in France: The World War I Diary of Maude Frances Essig," *Indiana Magazine of History,* 82:37–68, 1986.

Secondary Sources

Adams, Michael C. C., *Living Hell: The Dark Side of the Civil War*. Baltimore: Johns Hopkins University Press, 2014.

Adrian, E. D., and Yealland, L. R., "The Treatment of Some Common War Neuroses," *Lancet,* 189:867–872, 1917.

Arendt, Hannah, *Eichmann in Jerusalem:*

A Report on the Banality of Evil. New York: Viking, 1963.

Baer, W. S., "The Treatment of Chronic Osteomyelitis with the Maggot (larva of the blow fly)," *Journal of Bone and Joint Surgery,* 13:438–475, 1931.

Bankert, Marianne, *Watchful Care: A History of America's Nurse Anesthetists.* New York: Continuum, 1989.

Bardenheuer, V., *The Uses of Permanent Extension: Subcutaneous and Compound Fractures and Dislocations of the Extremities and Their Consequences.* New York: Stechert, 1889.

Barry, John M., *The Great Influenza: The Epic Story of the Deadliest Plague in History.* New York: Viking, 2004.

Baskett, Thomas F., "William O'Shaughnessy, Thomas Latta and the Origins of Intravenous Saline," *Resuscitation,* 55:231–234, 2002.

Bellafaire, Judith, and Graf, Mercedes Herrera, *Women Doctors in War.* College Station: Texas A&M University Press, 2009.

Bliss, Michael, *Harvey Cushing: A Life in Surgery.* Oxford: Oxford University Press, 2005.

Bond, Earl D., *Thomas W. Salmon—Psychiatrist.* New York: Norton, 1950.

Bornstein, Max, "Aids in the Use of Dakin-Carrel Treatment," *Journal of the American Medical Association,* 70:1820, 1918.

Bottorff, J. L., *Nurse-Patient Interaction: Observations of Touch.* Unpublished doctoral dissertation, University of Alberta, 1992.

Bristow, Nancy K., *American Pandemic: The Lost Worlds of the 1918 Influenza Epidemic.* Oxford: Oxford University Press, 2012.

Brock, Thomas D., *Robert Koch: A Life in Medicine and Bacteriology.* Washington, D.C.: ASM, 1998 [1988].

Brown, Edward, "Between Cowardice and Insanity: Shell Shock and the Legitimation of the Neuroses in Great Britain." In: Everett Mendelsohn, et al., eds., *Science, Technology and the Military.* Dordrecht: Kluwer, 1989, 323–345.

Brundage, John F., and Shanks, G. Dennis, "Deaths from Bacterial Pneumonia during 1918–19 Influenza Pandemic," *Emerging Infectious Diseases,* 14:1193–1199, 2008.

Bundy, Elizabeth Rosanna, *Surgical Nursing in War.* Phila: Blakiston, 1917.

Byerly, Carol R., *Fever of War: The Influenza Epidemic in the U.S. Army during World War I.* New York: New York University Press, 2005.

Carrel, A., and Dehelly, G., *The Treatment of Infected Wounds,* trans. Herbert Child. New York: Hoeber, 1917.

Carter, A., and Sanderson, H., "The Use of Touch in Nursing Practice," *Nurs. Standard,* 9:31–35, 1995.

Charles, Daniel, *Master Mind: The Rise and Fall of Fritz Haber, the Nobel Laureate Who Launched the Age of Chemical Warfare.* New York: HarperCollins, 2005.

Chase, Julia A. Houghton, *Mary A. Bickerdyke, "Mother": The Life Story of One who, as Wife, Mother, Army Nurse, Pension Agent and City Missionary, has Touched the Heights and Depths of Human Life.* Lawrence, KS: Journal Publishing House, 1896

Chomel, Marie, and Anselm, *Red Cross Chapter at Work.* Indianapolis: Hollenbeck, 1920.

Cirillo, Vincent J., *Bullets and Bacilli: The Spanish-American War and Military Medicine.* New Brunswick: Rutgers University Press, 2004.

Cobbs, Elizabeth, *The Hello Girls: America's First Women Soldiers.* Cambridge: Harvard University Press, 2017.

Cosnett, J. E., "The Origins of Intravenous Fluid Therapy," *Lancet,* 333:768–771, 1989.

Crathern, Alice Tarbell, *In Detroit Courage was the Fashion: The Contribution of Women to the Development of Detroit from 1701 to 1951.* Detroit: Wayne State, University Press, 1953.

Crile, George, *An Autobiography,* vol. 1, ed. Grace Crile. Phila: Lippincott, 1947.

Crosby, Alfred W., *America's Forgotten Pandemic: The Influenza of 1918,* 2nd ed. Cambridge: Cambridge University Press, 2003 [1989].

Crosby, Alfred W., *Epidemic and Peace, 1918*. Westport, CT: Greenwood, 1976.

Cushing, Harvey, *From a Surgeon's Journal, 1915–1918*. Boston: Little, Brown, 1936.

Dakin, Henry Drysdale, and Dunham, Edward Kellogg, *A Handbook on Antiseptics*. New York: Macmillan, 1917.

Dale, Charlotte, *Raising Professional Confidence: The Influence of the Anglo- Boer War (1899–1902) on the Development and Recognition of Nursing as a Profession*. Unpublished dissertation, University of Manchester, 2014.

Dale, Charlotte, "The Social Exploits and Behaviour of Nurses During the Anglo-Boer War, 1899–1902," in Helen Sweet and Sue Hawkins, eds., *Colonial Caring: A History of Colonial and Post-Colonial Nursing*. Manchester: Manchester University Press, 2015.

D'Antonio, Patricia, *American Nursing: A History of Knowledge, Authority, and the Meaning of Work*. Baltimore: John Hopkins University Press, 2010.

D'Arby, Louise B., "The Hospital X-Ray Nurse," *American Journal of Nursing*, 17:488–490, 1917.

Debue-Barazer, Christine, "La gangrène gazeuse pendant la Première Guerre mondiale (Front occidental)," *Annales de Démographie Historique*, 1[103]:51–70, 2002.

Deming, Dorothy, "Influenza—1918: Reliving the Great Epidemic," *American Journal of Nursing*, 57:1308–1309, 1957.

Deutsch, Hermann B., *Rudolph Matas: A Biography of One of the Great Pioneers in Surgery*. New York: Doubleday, 1960.

Dock, Lavinia L., et al., *History of the American Red Cross*. New York: Macmillan, 1922.

Dunne, J. S., "Notes on Surgical Work in a General Hospital—With Special Reference to the Carrel-Dakin Method of Treatment," *British Medical Journal*, 2:283–284, 1918.

Ebel, Jonathan, *Faith in the Fight: Religion and the American Soldier in the Great War*. Princeton: Princeton University Press, 2010.

Editorial, "American Nurses in Japan," *British Medical Journal*, 1:963–964, 1905.

Editorial, "Gas in Warfare," *Boston Medical and Surgical Journal*, 192:1024-1025, 1925.

Editorial, "She Helps the Wounded," *The Woman Citizen: The Woman's Journal*, 1:431, 3 November 1917.

Editorial, "War Gas Poisoning," *British Medical Journal*, 2:138–139, 1918.

Editorial, s.n., *The Biblical World*, 49:137–138, March, 1917.

Estabrooks, C. A., "Touch in Nursing Practice: A Historical Perspective: 1900- 1920," *Journal of Nursing History*, 2:33–49, 1987.

Estabrooks, C. A., and Morse, J. M., "Toward a Theory of Touch: The Touching Process and Acquiring a Touching Style," *Journal of Advanced Nursing*, 17:448–456, 1992.

Fairchild, Julie, *Making Room in the Clinic: Nurse Practitioners and the Evolution of Modern Health Care*. New Brunswick: Rutgers, 2008.

Falzeder, Ernest, and Brabant, Eva, eds., *The Correspondence of Sigmund Freud and Sandor Ferenczi, volume 2, 1914–1919*. Cambridge: Harvard University Press, 1996.

Fatović-Ferenčić, Stella, and Pećina, Mark, "The Balkan Beam—Florschütz Frame and its Use During the Great War," *International Orthopaedics*, 38:2209–2213, 2009.

Faust, Drew Gilpin Faust, *This Republic of Suffering: Death and the American Civil War*. New York: Random House, 2008.

Fitzgerald, Alice, "To Nurses Preparing for Active Service," *American Journal of Nursing*, 18:188–191, 1917.

Forsyth, David, "Functional Nerve Disease and the Shock of Battle," *Lancet*, 185:1399–1403, 1915.

Frantz, Ann K., "Clara Barton in the Spanish-American War," *American Journal of Nursing*, 98:39–41, 1998.

Freitas, L., "Historical Roots and Future Perspectives Related to Nursing Ethics," *Journal of Professional Nursing,* 197–205, 1990.

Gabriel, Richard A., *Between Flesh and Steel: A History of Military Medicine from the Middle Ages to the War in Afghanistan.* Washington, D.C.: Potomac, 2013.

Gamble, Richard, *The War for Righteousness: Progressive Christianity, the Great War, and the Rise of the Messianic Nation.* Wilmington, DE: ISI, 2003.

Gavin, Lettie, *American Women in World War I.* Niwot: University Press of Colorado, 1997.

Goldman, Leon, and Cullen, Glenn E., "Some Medical Aspects of Chemical Warfare Agents," *Journal of the American Medical Association,* 114:2200–2204, 1940.

Goldsmith, M., *A Report on Hospital Gangrene, Erysipelas: As Observed in the Departments of the Ohio and the Cumberland, with Cases Appended, and Pyemia,* published by permission of the surgeon General U.S.A. Louisville: Bradley & Gilbert, 1863.

Goostray, Sheila, "Mary Adelaide Nutting," *American Journal of Nursing* 58:1524–1529, 1958.

Graf, Mercedes H., *On the Field of Mercy: Women Medical Volunteers from the Civil War to the First World War.* Amherst, New York: Humanity Books, 2010.

Graf, Mercedes H., "Women Nurses in the Spanish-American War," *Minerva,* 19:3–19, 2001.

Grassberger, Martin, and Fleischmann, Wim, "The Biobag—A New Device for the Application of Medicinal Maggots." *Dermatology* (Basel), 204:306, 2002.

Groch-Begley, Hannah, "The Forgotten Female Shell-Shock Victims of World War I." *The Atlantic,* September 8, 2014.

Hallett, Christine, *Containing Trauma: Nursing Work in the First World War.* Manchester: Manchester University Press, 2009.

Hallett, Christine, *Nurses of Passchendaele: Caring for the Wounded of the Ypres Campaigns, 1914–1918.* South Yorkshire: Pen & Sword, 2017.

Hallett, Christine, *Veiled Warriors: Allied Nurses of the First World War.* Oxford: Oxford University Press, 2014.

Harden, Victoria A. Harden, *Inventing the NIH: Federal Biomedical Research Policy,1887–1937.* Baltimore: Johns Hopkins University Press, 1986.

Harrington, Ralph, "On the Tracks of Trauma: Railway Spine Reconsidered," *Social History of Medicine,* 16:209–223, 2003.

Hasegawa, Guy R., "Proposals for Chemical Weapons during the American Civil War," *Military Medicine,* 173:499–506, 2008.

Hine, Darlene Clark, *Black Women in White: Racial Conflict and Cooperation in the Nursing Profession, 1890–1950.* Bloomington: Indiana University Press, 1989.

Hinkson, De Haven, "Medical Aspect of Gas Warfare," *Journal of the National Medical Association,* 12:1–6, 1920.

Hirshfeld, Samuel, Hyman, Harold Thomas, and Wanger, Justine, "Influence of Velocity on the Response to Intravenous Injections," *Archives of Internal Medicine,* 47:259–287, 1931.

History of the Pennsylvania Hospital Unit (Base Hospital No. 10, USA). New York: Hoeber, 1921.

Howe, Mark A., comp., *The Occasional Speeches of Justice Oliver Wendell Holmes, Jr.* Cambridge: Harvard University Press, 1962.

Hyman, Harold Thomas, and Hirshfeld, Samuel, "Studies of Velocity and the Response to Intravenous Injections: III. Technic of the Intravenous Drip in Clinical Practice," *Journal of the American Medical Association,* 96:1221–1223, 1931.

Inder, W. S. *On Active Service with the S.J.A.B., South African War, 1899–1902.* Kendal: Atkinson and Pollitt, 1903.

Iyriboz, Yuruk, "A Recent Exposure to

Mustard Gas in the United States: Clinical Findings of a Cohort (n = 247) 6 Years after Exposure," *MedGenMed,* 6:4, 2004.

Janne, Anna C., "The Army School of Nursing," *American Journal of Nursing,* 19:179–184, 1918.

Jenkins, A. R., "The Padded Board Stretcher in the Treatment of Hip Disease and Various Traumata," *Annals of Surgery,* 8:105–109, 1888.

Jensen, Kimberly, *Mobilizing Minerva: American Women in the First World War.* Urbana: University of Illinois Press, 2008.

Johnson, W., and Rows, R.G., "Neurasthenia and War Neuroses," in *History of the Great War Based on Official Documents: Diseases of War,* Vol. 2. London: s.n., 1923.

Jones, Ann, *They Were Soldiers: How the Wounded Return from America's Wars—The Untold Story.* Chicago: Haymarket, 2013.

Jones, Edgar, "Historical Approaches to Post-Combat Disorders," *Philosophical Transactions of the Royal Society of Britain,* 361:533–542, 2006.

Jones, Edgar, and Wessely, Simon, "War Syndromes: The Impact of Culture on Medically Unexplained Symptoms," *Medical History,* 49:55–78, 2005.

Jones, Marian Moser, *The American Red Cross: From Clara Barton to the New Deal.* Baltimore: Johns Hopkins University Press, 2013.

Kalisch, Philip A., "Heroines of '98: Female Army Nurses in the Spanish-American War," *Nursing Research,* 24:411–429, 1975.

Keeling, Arlene W., "'Alert to the Necessities of the Emergency': U.S. Nursing during the 1918 Influenza Pandemic," *Public Health Reports,* 125(suppl. 3) 2010.

Keen, W. W., *The Treatment of War Wounds.* Phila: Saunders, 1917.

Keene, Jennifer D., *World War I: The American Soldier Experience.* Lincoln: University of Nebraska Press, 2011 [2006].

Kennedy, David M., *Over Here: The First World War and American Society.* Oxford: Oxford University Press, 2004 [1980].

Kinder, John, *Paying with Their Bodies: American War and the Problem of the Disabled Veteran.* Chicago: University of Chicago Press, 2015.

Koch, Bruce Evan, "Surgeon-Nurse Anesthetist Collaboration Advanced Surgery between 1889 and 1950," *Anethesia-Analgesia,* 12:653–662, 2015.

Kohut, Heinz, *How Does Analysis Cure?* ed. Arnold Goldberg with the collaboration of Paul E. Stepansky. Chicago: University of Chicago Press, 1984.

Kolata, Gina, *Flu: The Story of the Great Influenza Pandemic of 1918 and the Search for the Virus That Caused It.* New York: Farrar, Straus and Giroux, 2011.

Kuhn, Thomas, *The Essential Tension: Selected Studies in Tradition and Change.* Chicago: University of Chicago Press, 1977.

Kuhn, Thomas, *The Structure of Scientific Revolutions.* Chicago: University of Chicago Press, 1970.

Lenhart, M. K., and Tuorinsky, S. D., eds., *Medical Aspects of Chemical Warfare.* Washington, D.C.: Office of the Surgeon General, 2008.

Liebenau, Jonathan, *Medical Science and Medical Industry: The Formation of the American Pharmaceutical Industry.* Baltimore: Johns Hopkins University Press, 1987.

Linker, Beth, *War's Waste: Rehabilitation in World War I America.* Chicago: University of Chicago Press, 2011.

MacFarlane, Gwyn, *Alexander Fleming: The Man and the Myth.* Cambridge: Harvard University Press, 1984.

Macleod, A. D., "Shell Shock, Gordon Homes and the Great War," *Journal of the Royal Society of Medicine,* 97:86–89, 2004.

Makita, Yoshiya, "Professional Angels at War: The United States Army Nursing Service and Changing Ideals of Nursing at the Turn of the Twentieth Century," *Japanese Journal of American Studies*, 24:2013, 67- 86.

Maranda, Eric Laurent, et al., "Chemical Warfare's Most Notorious Agent against the Skin," *JAMA Dermatology*, 152:933, 2016.

McCall, Susan C., "Lessons Learned by Army Nurses in Combat: A Historical Review," Individual Study Project (unclassified), 15 April 1993, Army War College, Carlisle Barracks, PA.

Medical Department of the United States Army in The World War, Volume II: Administration American Expeditionary Forces, prepared under the direction of Maj. Gen. M. W. Ireland, by Colonel Joseph H. Ford. Washington, D.C.: U.S. Government Printing Office, 1927.

Meyers, Charles S., *Shell Shock in France, 1914–1918, Based on a War Diary*. Cambridge: Cambridge University Press, 1940.

Morantz, Regina, "Feminism, Professionalism, and Germs: The Thought of Mary Putnam Jacobi and Elizabeth Blackwell," *American Quarterly*, 34:459–478, 1982.

Morantz-Sanchez, Regina, *Sympathy and Science: Women Physicians in American Medicine*. Chapel Hill: University of North Carolina Press, 1985.

More, Ellen S., "'A Certain Restless Ambition': Women Physicians and World War I," *American Quarterly*, 41:1989, 636–660.

Morens, David M., et al., "Role of Bacterial Pneumonia as a Cause of Death in Pandemic Influenza: Implications for Pandemic Influenza Preparedness," *Journal of Infectious Diseases*, 198:962–970, 2008.

Mulaik, J. S., et al., "Patients' Perceptions of Nurses' Use of Touch," *Western Journal of Nursing Research*, 13:306–323, 1991.

Mumcuoglu, Kosta Y., "Clinical Applications for Maggots in Wound Care," *American Journal of Clinical Dermatology*, 4:219–227, 2001.

Neiberg, Michael S., *The Path to War: How the First World War Created Modern America*. New York: Oxford University Press, 2016.

Nightingale, Florence, *Notes on Nursing: What Nursing Is, What Nursing Is Not*. New York: Appleton, 1860 [1859].

Oates, Stephen B., *A Woman of Valor: Clara Barton and the Civil War*. New York: Free Press, 1994.

O'Neill, Teresa M., *"I Wanted to Do Something for the Country": Experiences of Military Nurses in World War II*. Unpublished doctoral dissertation, School of Nursing, University of Miami, 2003.

Parsons, Marion G., "Some Points in the Nursing of a Fractured Femur in the Home," *American Journal of Nursing*, 9:104–111, 1908.

Pavic, Roman, "Prof. Vatroslav Florschütz and the Balkan Beam Frame," *Injury*, 42:225–226, 2011.

Pierce, Gerald J., *Public and Private Voices: The Typhoid Fever Experience at Camp Thomas*. Unpublished doctoral dissertation, Department of History, Georgia State University, 2007.

Pilcher, E. M., and Hull, A. J., "The Treatment of Wounds by Flavine," *British Medical Journal*, i2908:172, 1918.

Pinsker, Henry, et al., *Dynamic Supportive Psychotherapy: Handbook of Short-Term Dynamic Psychotherapy*. New York: Basic Books, 1991.

Pope, Georgina Fane, "Nursing in South Africa During the Boer War, 1899–1900," *American Journal of Nursing*, 3:10–14, 1902.

Prothero, Stephen, *American Jesus: How the Son of God Became a National Hero*. New York: Farrar, Straus & Giroux, 2003.

Pryor, Elizabeth Brown, *Clara Barton: Professional Angel*. Philadelphia: University of Pennsylvania Press, 1988.

Ramon, Martin, "Anesthesia at Base Hospital No. 5," presented at the 9th International Symposium on the History of Anesthesia, Boston, MA, 2017.

Read, C. Stanford, *Military Psychiatry in Peace and War*. London: Lewis, 1920.

Reverby, Susan M., *Ordered to Care: The Dilemma of American Nursing, 1850–*

1945. Cambridge: Cambridge University Press, 1987.

Robb, Isabel Hampton, *Nursing Ethics.* Cleveland: Koeckert, 1900.

Robb, Isabel Hampton, *Nursing: Its Principles and Practice, for Hospital and Private Use.* Phila: Saunders, 1893.

Roberts, John B., "Treatment of the Lower End of the Humerus and of the Base of the Radius," *Annals of Surgery,* 16:1–41, 1892.

Robinson, Frances, "Maggot Therapy for Wound Healing," *Wound Care,* 12 February 2010, 28–29.

Rosen, George, "Nostalgia: A 'Forgotten' Psychological Disorder," *Psychological Medicine,* 5:340–354, 1975.

Russell, Edmund, *War and Nature: Fighting Humans and Insects with Chemical Weapons from World War I to Silent Spring.* Cambridge: Cambridge University Press, 2001.

Ryle, J. A., "Discussion on Gas Poisoning," *Proceedings of the Royal Society of Medicine,* 13 (war section):47–48, 1920.

Salmon, Thomas W., *The Care and Treatment of Mental Diseases and War Neuroses ("Shell Shock") in the British Army.* New York: National Committee for Mental Hygiene, 1917.

Salvi, Andrea Emilio, et al., "The Invention of the Balkan Beam Frame," *Injury,* 40:1237–1238, 2009.

Sandelowski, Margaret, *Devices and Desires: Gender, Technology, and American Nursing.* Chapel Hill: University of North Carolina Press, 2000.

Sarnecky, Mary, *A History of the U.S. Army Nurse Corps.* Philadelphia: University of Pennsylvania Press, 1999.

Schultz, Jane E., *Women at the Front: Hospital Workers in Civil War America.* Chapel Hill: University of North Carolina Press, 2004.

Senn, Nicholas, *Medico-Surgical Aspects of the Spanish American War.* Chicago: AMA Press, 1900.

Shanks, G. Dennis, et al., "Low But Highly Variable Mortality among Nurses and Physicians during the Influenza Pandemic of 1918–1919," *Influenza and other Respiratory Viruses,* 5:213–219, 2011.

Shephard, Ben, *A War of Nerves: Soldiers and Psychiatrists in the Twentieth Century.* Cambridge: Harvard University Press, 2001.

Sherman, Ronald A. "Maggot Therapy Takes Us Back to the Future of Wound Care: New and Improved Maggot Therapy for the 21st Century," *Journal of Diabetes Science & Technology,* 3:336–339, 2009.

Sherman, William O'Neill, "The Abortive Treatment of Wound Infection: Carrel's Method—Dakin's Solution." *Journal of the American Medical Association,* 69:185–192, 1917.

Sinclair, Rodney D., and Ryan, Terence J., "A Great War for Antiseptics," *Australasian Journal of Dermatology,* 34:115–118, 1993.

Smith, Helen Zenna, *Not so Quiet...Stepdaughters of War.* New York: Feminist Press of CUNY: 1989 [1930].

Stagner, Annessa C., "Healing the Soldier, Restoring the Nation: Representations of Shell Shock in the USA During and After the First World War," *Journal of Contemporary History,* 49:255–274, 2014.

Starns, Penny, *Nurses at War, Women on the Frontline, 1939–45* Gloucestershire: Sutton, 2000.

Stepansky, Paul E., *Freud, Surgery, and the Surgeons.* New York: Routledge, 1999.

Stepansky, Paul E., *In the Hands of Doctors: Touch and Trust in Medical Care.* Santa Barbara: Praeger, 2016.

Stepansky, Paul E., *Psychoanalysis at the Margins.* New York: Other Press, 2009.

Stoltzenberg, Detrich, *Fritz Haber: Chemist, Nobel Laureate, German Jew.* Lexington, MA: Plunkett Lake, 2015 [1994].

Sullivan, Harry Stack, *The Interpersonal Theory of Psychiatry,* ed. Helen Swick Perry and Mary Ladd Gawel. New York: Norton, 1953.

Thatcher, Virginia S., *History of Anesthe-*

sia, with Emphasis on the Nurse Specialist. Phila: Lippincott, 1953.

Thompson, George, "Battlefield Medicine: The American Response to Gas
Gangrene on the Western Front." Unpublished manuscript, Department of
the History and Philosophy of Medicine School of Medicine, University of
Kansas Medical Center, s.a.

Tomblin, Barbara Brooks, G.I. Nightingales: The Army Nurse Corps in World
War II. Lexington: University of Kentucky Press, 1996.

Tucker, Holly, Blood Work: A Tale of
Medicine and Murder in the Scientific
Revolution. New York: Norton, 2012.

Vaughan, Victor C., A Doctor's Memories.
Indianapolis: Bobbs-Merrill, 1926.

Viets, Henry, "Shell-Shock: A Digest of
the English Literature," Journal of
the American Medical Association,
19:1779–1786, 1917.

Vincent, Jean-Louis, and Hall, Jesse B.,
Encyclopedia of Intensive Care Medicine, Berlin: Springer-Verlag, 2012.

Volk, Katherine. Buddies in Budapest.
Los Angeles: Kellaway-Ide, 1936.

Vuic, Kara Dixon, Officer, Nurse, Woman:
The Army Nurse Corps in the Vietnam
War. Baltimore: Johns Hopkins Univer-
sity Press, 2011.

Weiss, S. J., "The Language of Touch,"
Nursing Research, 28:76–80, 1979.

Weiss, S. J., "Psychophysiological Effects
of Caregiver Touch on Incidence of
Cardiac Dysrhythmia," Heart Lung,
15:494–505, 1986.

Whitaker, Iain S., et al., "Larval therapy
from Antiquity to the Present Day:
Mechanisms of Action, Clinical Applications and Future Potential," Postgraduate Medical Journal, 83:409–
413, 1980.

Winnicott, D. W., The Maturational
Processes and the Facilitating Environment: Studies in the Theory of Emotional Development. New York: International Universities Press, 1965.

Wood, John, "On the Employment of
Double Extension in Cases of Disease
and Injuries of the Spine and Pelvic
Joints," British Medical Journal,
1(1014):837–838, 1880.

Wright, A. E., "An Address on Wound Infections; and on Some New Methods
for the Study of the Various Factors
Which Come into Consideration in
Their Treatment," Proceedings of the
Royal Society of Medicine, 8:41–86,
1915.

Yealland, Lewis R., Hysterical Disorders
of Warfare. London: Macmillan, 1918.

Zeiger, Susan, In Uncle Sam's Service:
Women Workers with the American Ex-
peditionary Force, 1917–1919. Ithaca:
Cornell University Press, 1999.

Index